Growing Healthy

Teresa Mitchell

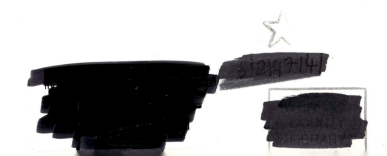

Note for Librarians: A cataloguing record for this book is available from Library and Archives Canada at www.collectionscanada.ca/amicus/index-e.html

ISBN 1-4251-0067-8

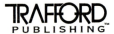

PUBLISHING™

Offices in Canada, USA, Ireland and UK

Book sales for North America and international:
Trafford Publishing, 6E–2333 Government St.,
Victoria, BC V8T 4P4 CANADA
phone 250 383 6864 (toll-free 1 888 232 4444)
fax 250 383 6804; email to orders@trafford.com

Book sales in Europe:
Trafford Publishing (UK) Limited, 9 Park End Street, 2nd Floor
Oxford, UK OX1 1HH UNITED KINGDOM
phone +44 (0)1865 722 113 (local rate 0845 230 9601)
facsimile +44 (0)1865 722 868; info.uk@trafford.com

Order online at:
trafford.com/06-1824

10 9 8 7 6 5 4 3 2

GROWING HEALTHY
T. H. Mitchell MD MRCPUK FRCPI FFPM ABIM

About the author

Dr. Mitchell has a lifetime of experience in medicine. She is a specialist in general medicine, diabetes, endocrinology and metabolism who has also worked in chemical pathology, toxicology, clinical pharmacology and regulatory medicine. She is a graduate of Trinity College, Dublin with honours degrees in Physical Chemistry and Medicine and a Master's degree in Molecular Medicine. She has worked in Ireland, Britain, USA and Canada and has lectured widely in medicine and regulatory medicine including molecular medicine. She is a Fellow of the Royal College of Physicians of Ireland. She holds membership of the UK Royal College of Physicians and American College of Physicians, is Board Certified in Internal Medicine from the USA and was awarded Fellowship in Pharmaceutical Medicine by distinction, by the Royal College of Pharmaceutical Physicians of London. She recently received a Diploma in Management for Medical Doctors from the Royal College of Surgeons in Ireland and the Institute of Public Administration.

About the book

The book is intended for anyone who wants to prevent illness by adopting a sensible lifestyle. Lifestyle affects you, your home and your work and leisure environment. For each of us there is an interplay between the individual and his environment. The way each of these exerts its effect determines the future.

This book is dedicated to Bridget Mitchell

Contents

Glossary

AAT deficiency	Alpha-1 antitrypsin deficiency
ADHD	Attention Deficit Hyperactivity Disorder
A & E	Accident and Emergency
AIDS	Acquired immune deficiency syndrome
Alopecia	Loss of hair on the scalp
Analgesic	Painkiller
Androgens	Male hormones
Autoimmune	The body reacts against itself.
BCG	Bacille Calmette-Guérin
Binge	Prolonged use over a short time
BMI	Body Mass Index
	= body weight in kilogram divided by (height in metre)^2
	healthy range 19-25
	obese $\geq$ 30
	1 pound = 0.45kg
	1 foot = 0.3metre
Bronchitis	Inflammation of the airways
CCTV	Closed circuit TV
Cervix	Neck of womb
CFS	Chronic Fatigue Syndrome
Cholecystectomy	Removal of the gall bladder
Colon	Large bowel
Diabetes mellitus	'Sugar diabetes'
DNA	Deoxyribonucleic acid
DVT	Deep venous thrombosis
ECG	Electrocardiogram
Emphysema	A condition where the lung air cells lose their elasticity
Enzyme	A protein which influences chemical processes in the body
EPA	Environmental Protection Agency
EU	European Union
Foetus	Unborn baby
Fracture	Break in the bone

GAA	Gaelic Athletic Association
GM	Genetically modified
Halitosis	Bad breath
Herpes zoster	Shingles
HIV	Human immunodeficiency virus
Hirsutism	Excessive hair growth on the face and body
HSE	Health Service Executive
Hormone	A secretion of the endocrine or ductless glands
IARC	The International Agency for Research on Cancer
IBS	Irritable bowel syndrome
Impotence	Inability to get an erection
IQ	Intelligence quotient
Larynx	Voice-box
LSD	Lysergic acid diethylamide
ME	Myalgic encephalomyelitis
MMR vaccine	Measles, mumps, rubella vaccine
MRSA	Methicillin-resistant Staphylococcus aureus
MS	Multiple sclerosis
MSH	Melanocyte stimulating hormone
Neurotransmitter	Transmits signals between brain cells
Nocturia	Getting up at night to pass urine
NSC	National Safety Council
Obesity	BMI $\geq$ 30
	Waist size > 35 inches in females, >40 inches in males
	1 inch = 2.54cm
OCD	Obsessive-compulsive disorder
Oesophagus	Gullet
PABA	Para-aminobenzoic acid
Palpitations	Rapid heart beat
PCBs	Polychlorinated biphenyls
PCOS	Polycystic ovary syndrome
PCR	Polymerase chain reaction

PKU	Phenylketonuria
Promiscuity	Indiscriminate sexual relations
PSA	Prostatic-specific antigen
Rectum	End of large bowel
RNA	Ribonucleic acid
RPII	Radiological Protection Institute of Ireland
RTA	Road Traffic Accident
Rubella	German measles
SAD	Seasonal affective disorder
SCDS	Sudden cardiac death syndrome
SIDS	Sudden infant death syndrome
SLE	Systemic lupus erythematosus
Sterility	Inability to have children
Sublingual tablet	Tablet which dissolves under the tongue
TB	Tuberculosis
TENS	Transcutaneous electrical nerve stimulation
Teratogenic	Deforming birth defect
Uterus	Womb
Varicella	Chickenpox
Venereal disease	Disease communicated by sexual intercourse
Virus	Micro-organism
WHO	World Health Organization

Introduction

Y ou do not have to study medicine to keep healthy. You do need to know the facts about food, exercise and health promotion. Only you can keep yourself healthy. Health is our biggest wealth. Healthy citizens are more productive citizens. Ireland has one of the youngest populations in the EU however it is not one of the healthiest populations. Government leaflets have tried to promote awareness of health issues and more people are becoming involved in their own health care. Unfortunately, the message does not reach all, particularly those underprivileged in our society who may not have the ability to read. There are huge gaps in health, mental health and education. In 2004 literacy difficulties were found to be present in at least 25% of Irish adults. These problems cause people embarrassment and poor self-image since they continually need to make excuses to cover their inability to read and write. Poor communication is a barrier to health and there is a significant correlation between low literacy rates and poor health.

A recent study in the UK has indicated that the Irish in Britain are one of the unhealthiest of all ethnic groups. In the USA many young Irish people have been shown to lack coping skills. These young men and women are often forced into or choose unsuitable employment, starting a spiral downwards into depression and cocaine abuse. Even more worrying are the reports of single well-educated Irish women in the USA who are working in low-paid jobs, have low self–esteem and often end up in abusive relationships. Lack of emotional intelligence may be responsible for these situations and probably reflects both inadequate parental and school guidance.

Lifestyle today may be increasing depression and stress. Alcohol and drug abuse, road traffic accidents (RTAs), unintentional work-related and home injuries, and suicide are far too common in Irish society. Clearly there is something wrong with a society which seems to have gross insecurity about itself. In the 1960s the annual suicide rate was 64 and suicide in men was rare outside of Dublin. Figures for 2003 were 444, many of these in rural areas with spiralling levels of suicide in certain parts of the country. 399 deaths occurred on Irish roads from January to mid-December 2005 with alcohol excess and speeding being major contributors to this figure. Binge drinking rates amongst Irish women are the highest in the EU. While one fifth of the population never drink alcohol, almost 50% of drivers have had a drink before driving. Ireland's alcohol consumption has doubled since 1970. In Ireland the average household spends Euro1,675 per year on alcohol. Longer drinking hours have boosted binge drinking, incidence of reported rape and violence. Alcohol is destroying young, middle-aged and elderly lives. Venereal disease is increasing significantly in Ireland. Although Ireland has now got an average 32 hour week, less than half of households have a pet. Ireland puts down more dogs than most other EU countries and in itself this can have a negative impact on national life.

At least 15% of Irish people are seriously overweight. Obesity is overtaking smoking as the leading cause of preventable death. Obesity causes people to get premature disease of the heart, joints and brain and increases the risk of cancer. Obesity also leads in many cases to diabetes mellitus.

Prematurity is the leading cause of infant death and premature births at 37 weeks or less have risen in several EU countries including Ireland, possibly because the mothers are getting older and heavier. In 2005 the average birth weight in Ireland was found to be around 4.1kg compared to 3.4kg in 1995. This means that a considerable proportion of newborn babies are heavier than 4.1kg, possibly leading to heavier adolescents. Mothers with babies of 4.1kg or greater are at increased risk themselves of getting diabetes. As many as nine babies in every thousand in Ireland may be born with health problems due to alcohol, which can later result in Attention Deficit Hyperactivity Disorder (ADHD) and poor coordination. Some psychiatrists question the existence of a medical condition called ADHD. While there are no medical tests for ADHD, it probably does exist as a pathological condition however it must not be over-diagnosed on the basis of bad behaviour alone.

Ireland has the fourth highest number of asthmatics per population in the world with 15% of children suffering with asthma and 20% of school-going children have symptoms consistent with asthma. Rates for lung cancer in Irish women are double the EU average and there are approximately 900 deaths per year from bowel cancer. Mouth cancer possibly due to binge drinking is rising steadily amongst Irish women. Our intermediate care strategy for those who are sick has not been adequate. Travel is a major issue for patients. The positive effects of treatment are lessened by the tedium of travel over long distances. Communities must have a say in local health support.

The earlier you begin the better, but it is never too late to become informed about your health. Simple concepts must be grasped. Smoking, lack of exercise and poor nutrition account for one in three premature deaths. Smoking strongly reduces the chances of surviving from 40 to 70 years of age by increasing the risk of heart and lung disease. Smoking exposes children to toxins which may cause lifelong problems. Lack of exercise and poor nutrition lead to obesity. In children, regular 'fast food' may lead to lack of attainment of real potential, and to hyperactivity. While sensible eating and regular exercise is important it is essential to keep mentally active as well. While learning, the brain is challenged. The phrase 'Use it or lose it' is particularly applicable to the brain. A mind challenged by reading is likely to remain alert while an unchallenged brain stops learning and may deteriorate.

Overemphasis on material values must not be allowed to push people towards violence, suicide, alcohol and drugs. Drug abuse or alcohol excess may have catastrophic acute and chronic effects on the brain particularly the immature brain of a teenager. Sports organizations must stop promoting alcohol. Advertisements must stop portraying Ireland as a 'Big pint and a round of drinks'. The 'prattle and craic' is a trifle passé! Parents must take preventive action and not allow their children to harm themselves or others due to excess alcohol. If alcohol-induced damage to person and property is to be reduced then early education and adequately enforced political measures will be necessary.

The environment has an important role in health. Pathogenic organisms seek new hosts when their habitat is destroyed by cutting down trees or by dumping. We must strive for clean air, absence of smoking, unpolluted rivers with absence of dumping, and a surrounding of non-vandalized trees. It is important to live and to work in a clean environment, to enjoy leisure time and not to confuse alcohol excess with culture and enjoyment. If your job, done to the best of your ability, is not working for you, change it now.

While the chief purpose of our Health Service is to treat illness, since health resources are finite and will always be limited, the importance of avoiding preventable disease must be stressed. A large percentage of people attending the Accident and Emergency (A & E) Department have medical problems. A lot of these problems can be prevented. Try and stay out of hospital by adopting a healthier lifestyle. The national emphasis on alcohol as part of Irish culture must change with the aim of reducing alcohol consumption, RTAs, sexual disease and suicide.

For all, exercise is the cornerstone and key to health promotion. In fact rising levels of obesity are probably due more to lack of exercise than to excess food consumption, however it is important to eat moderate portions of good quality food rather than large portions of processed food. In order to enhance our ability to be a healthy population in the future, the provision of adequate drug-free sports facilities, public swimming pools and inner city facilities must be encouraged. This is one of the most productive ways of preventing the downward spiral into drug use, unemployment and crime. It will also reduce obesity and diabetes and will more than compensate for initial resources deployed. Aggression in sport must however never be encouraged.

Although we have access to excellent food, uninformed consumers tend to accept big portions of high salt, high fat low quality processed food and the market caters for the customer's demands. To foresee the future one only has to look to the US where many of the present generation of Americans are obese following consumption of vast quantities of processed food and are likely to have a shorter life expectancy than their parents. To know the facts about exercise, diet and health promotion will empower you to prevent common illness such as heart disease, diabetes mellitus and cancer. In the twenty-five chapters that follow, general well-being, accident and disease prevention, and some aspects of common disease will be discussed. There is a beginning when you will be curious, a middle when you will feel interested and hopefully, a happy ending when you will feel that you are in charge and able to manage your health. For simplicity 'he/him' are used throughout. Obviously this can refer to male or female. It is noteworthy however that men die about six years younger than women and have higher death rates at all ages. Men generally seem to take health issues less seriously than women. However in the case of cancer of the lung, Irish women are rapidly catching up and in fact the rate of increase for this cancer is now higher in women than in men, because of smoking. Things that are obvious to one person may not be obvious to others. If you are worried about something, talk it through and ask questions. It is wise to ask questions about things that worry you because worry causes stress and excessive stress shortens life.

All parents must be empowered to educate their children. All children, regardless of any physical or mental disability, must have access to the best education possible. Better targeting of resources is needed to educate limited ability and special–needs pupils. Everyone has a unique personality which must be developed and nurtured. Since primary school education is the only education that some children can or wish to have, it must provide excellent basic education with an option at a later stage for further academia or practical skills. With good knowledge of computer systems gaps in numeracy and mathematics can be overcome. The key to better education involves smaller classes, better teaching, better attendance and better home and school discipline. Education must be the key to a better and healthier future for all. Educational and creative regeneration of culturally-deprived areas must take place. Efforts must be made to find local leaders who have the necessary kudos and ability to make things happen, to avoid alcohol and drug culture, to benefit everyone and improve social and mental health.

Key sentences: Health is our biggest wealth. Smoking, lack of exercise and poor nutrition account for one in three premature deaths. Binge drinking rates amongst Irish women are one of the highest in the EU. The importance of avoiding preventable disease must be stressed.

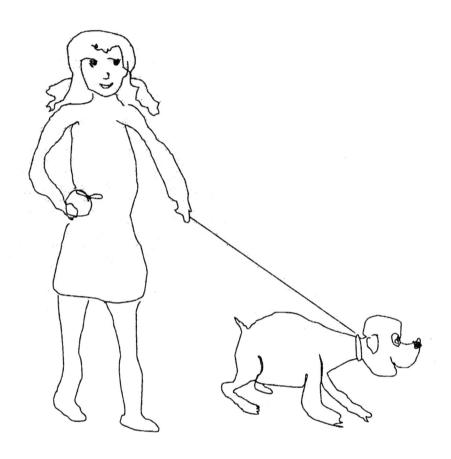

PREVENTION IS BETTER THAN CURE

1

The Beginning

George Bernard Shaw's wife Constance, left money to the Irish State for the purpose of educating Irish people. While at the time this was seen as somewhat insulting, similar benefactors and bequests today would benefit a lot of Irish people who have fallen out of the educational system. In 2000 the inequality in health between rich and poor was highlighted by the Director of the Institute of Public Health in Ireland. Literacy difficulties are highest amongst the poor and poorly educated. This means that they are not able to follow adequately the dosage instructions on a paracetamol packet, to understand what ingredients are on the label of the food products they are buying, or to fill in application forms. It is thus highly inappropriate, as highlighted by the media in 2004, that children from well-off families are getting one third of student grants. Paying money to school drop-outs to encourage them to attend courses is also of little use. To avail of education and rise out of poverty and alcohol and drug misuse, the environment must be stimulating and conducive to education. Adequate student grants must be redirected towards the poorest families and progress monitored and constantly reappraised. Education and access to education for all must be the Government objective. A renaissance in education with a much more varied curriculum is overdue. What child would not thrive if he excels at something, has a satisfying role in society and a sense of responsibility for himself?

While the Irish in Britain have made a vast contribution there, many of the homeless in the UK are from Ireland which reflects poorly on the Irish social services and educational system with its lack of coping skills. The Irish in Britain also form a significant proportion of the psychiatric admissions in the UK for alcoholism, depression and schizophrenia. While the Irish Government in recent years has made significant cash injections to UK-based psychotherapy services which serve the Irish community, better education and support in Ireland to prevent emotional or mental health problems in those choosing to emigrate might show long-term benefit.

Stress gives rise to unease, low productivity, increased risk taking leading to accidents, high sickness absence, addictive behaviour and mental health effects including suicide. A considerable number of Irish people suffer with panic attacks, with fears about health, anxiety and avoidance behaviour. These disorders occur more frequently in families with alcohol problems, in caffeine or cocaine addiction and in subjects with manic-depression. 'Hangovers' are responsible for a considerable loss of work days.

Television has created the impression of being able to 'have it all'. When this does not materialize, frustration sets in. In a rural area, inability to find local entertainment, public transport, or to pursue a hobby or a sport not linked to alcohol excess, or any form of social interaction apart from alcohol consumption in the local pub, all contribute to a feeling of inadequacy. The growing pressures to succeed at work, in educational attainment, social status and in love are stressing teenagers, adults and our pets. The pressure to be 'something' is putting impossible expectations upon children. Teenagers rob themselves of childhood by experimenting sexually because they feel this is the thing to do rather than what they actually want to do. Too much money in a society unused to money has caused poor discipline, binge drinking, and depression. Increasing stress, loneliness and lack of social or medical support for depression have all caused suicide rates to increase. Men may also feel that independent women are causing role reversal with men unsure of their role and status in society. There must be no stigma attached to those who seek treatment for psychiatric disorders, alcohol or substance abuse, however, the emphasis must be on disease prevention by moving away from the dysfunctional elements so prevalent in society today.

There are many reasons why people commit suicide. At-risk groups such as schizophrenic patients and subjects with either manic-depression or depression are more likely to attempt suicide. Suicide in one partner significantly increases the risk in the other and copy-cat suicide also occurs amongst teenagers. Drug and alcohol abuse are very important factors. When social status, other psychiatric disorders and alcohol dependence are controlled, there is a significant link between cannabis and suicide attempts. Suicide in all groups should be preventable. Although state-funded research projects to help reduce suicide have been established for some time, the suicide rate in Ireland, particularly in men, remains unacceptably high.

In the 1960s the annual suicide rate was 64 and suicide in men was rare outside of Dublin. Suicide now accounts for one third of all deaths in the 15-24 year age group. In 2003 there were 444 suicide deaths registered in Ireland, with the highest suicide rate for five years occurring in men 20-29 years old, many of these in rural areas with spiralling levels of suicide in certain parts of the country. This trend seems to be continuing with 194 suicides, 141 of which were male, in the first six months of 2004. Suicide is also increasing amongst women. The majority of subjects who self-harm admit that some form of support such as counselling or psychological help would be useful. A new vision for mental health in Ireland is needed. Better deployment of existing psychiatric resources should be commenced and a project that has apparently reduced the levels of self-harm, depression and suicide in Germany should be at least evaluated here since no national strategy has been successful. By contrast with Ireland the suicide rate for men in the UK has fallen to its lowest level for nearly 20 years, dropping almost 30% from its peak in 1998, so investigation of the UK strategy should be undertaken.

Lifestyle must be conducive to good health. A good public transport system and its use by commuters says a lot about a country's maturity and sophistication. Public transport needs to be of high calibre, treated with respect and be used where possible. In Ireland, excessive car and juggernaut use is blighting lives, wildlife and landscape. Mind and body

3

are often tired due to needless car use in our cities, causing gridlock and stress. In areas served by good public transport, fat children are still transported to school in cars. Although the average Irish worker does not work the longest hours compared with other EU countries, many appear to be suffering from 'burnout' leaving them in a constant state of stress in order to accumulate money for the children, for alcohol, for cigarettes, for cars and foreign holidays. Despite the evidence of sleep's important role in good health, sleep deprivation is common. Lack of sleep has been linked to obesity, diabetes, heart problems, psychiatric disorders and dementia and increases a person's chance of having an accident.

Many workers in the 25-50 age group are too busy to take lunch-breaks and end up regularly eating a fat-filled, salt-laden takeaway plus a sugar-filled drink, slumped over a desk. Some may eat nothing until evening time when excess food is eaten with copious alcohol. 'Heartburn' follows and then several tablets are used to correct this. A vicious circle is established. Potential sportsmen often show initial energy but seem to lack stamina and concentration possibly due to excess alcohol. Too many empty aspirations and emotional indulgence have perhaps dimmed the perspective of young people who are insecure and can look no further for excitement than binge drinking. Unsupervised foreign holidays after completing secondary school centre, in many cases, around excess alcohol consumption, loss of inhibition with vomiting and urination in public and exposure to sexual disease or risk of death by inhaling vomit or suffering an RTA. People need to pursue a less toxic style of enjoying themselves and sporting organizations need to reduce the drink culture.

In the last hundred years there has been a shift in disease pattern from infection to obesity. Serious fatness means a waist size greater than 35 inches (88 cm) in women and 40 inches (102 cm) in men. This arises by exercising less than one should and eating more than one needs. Obesity increases the risk of heart disease, diabetes and stroke. Diabetes, which can cause heart disease, blindness, kidney failure and gangrene of the toes, is increasing at an alarming rate throughout the world, particularly in western countries. This is mainly because people are using their cars excessively, are not walking enough, are eating too much and are getting fatter. Diabetes if unchecked will lower the increased life expectancy of the twenty-first century.

The aim must be to create awareness of the seriousness of being obese, and to empower all to do something about it. It is essential to prevent all non-obese individuals particularly children from becoming obese. One must not be obsessed by trying to achieve an ideal body weight. Rather achieve a stable weight than a fluctuating or steadily increasing weight. Reduce the crisps and the fizzy drinks. Convenience food is the easy option when life is busy. Parental emphasis must be on buying good quality food and not to offer second helpings. Time must be found for cooking the food and fast processed meals must not be consumed on a regular basis. If food does not have to travel far, it should contain fewer chemicals, fewer preservatives and fewer flavour and texture enhancers. Where possible buy local potatoes, carrots, strawberries, apples and salad rather than produce that has travelled many thousands of miles and therefore requires additives to keep it fresh. It is important to know the source of your food particularly meat and poultry. Animal welfare must also remain a strong consideration in food production.

Asthma probably 'runs in families' but it is exacerbated by house dust, smoking, air pollutants and certain foods. Ireland has one of the highest lung disease death rates in Europe. While lung cancer incidence in men less than 65 years is falling, in women, deaths from lung cancer are double the EU average due to increasing smoking rates. Children are therefore frequently and unfairly exposed to cigarette smoke. The unborn baby and newborn infant are also exposed to cigarette smoke which may cause lifelong problems. Smoking cessation would save a lot of ill-health, lives and money. The environment needs to be kept pure with avoidance of illegal dumping, illegal waste burning and smoking. By contrast with Ireland, the incidence of asthma has decreased in the UK, possibly because smoking has decreased in both men and women. It is important to remember that smoking and heart disease causes far more deaths in women than breast cancer.

One in twelve women might get breast cancer at some stage in life so early diagnosis is important. An EU study has shown that over the last ten years, breast cancer mortality for all women has dropped by 25% due possibly to increased awareness. This study also indicated that for

5

those women who participated in breast screening by mammography, the reduction in death rate was better, at 37%. While mammography may be more efficient in some women than others, it remains the best way of detecting breast cancer at an early stage. If these study results are valid in Ireland, it means that some women in the west and south of the country are dying because breast screening has not been available to detect their cancer early and allow suitable treatment. With the HSE policy of 'equality for all' this situation will have to change.

Irish people in Britain die earlier than the English or Welsh-born population or any other ethnic group apart from the Scots. Irish men have a greater risk of dying from cancer of the larynx (voice-box) than the general population. In the UK the Irish are identified as heavy alcohol drinkers regardless of whether individually they drink alcohol or not. They have a high rate of admission to psychiatric hospitals and an above average rate of suicide. The ill health also continues into the next two generations. The reason for the poor health is partly genetic but mainly environmental. Working long and unsociable hours for many years in the construction industry with inadequate health and safety regulations has perhaps taken its toll. Many of these workers have had poor social conditions, diet has been poor with lack of fruit and vegetable consumption, excessive alcohol consumption and very high smoking rates for men and women. Improved lifestyle, greater assertiveness and improved coping skills are necessary to avoid recurrence in the younger generation.

There are 1800 new cases of cancer of the colon and rectum in Ireland each year and approximately 900 annual deaths from these diseases. These cancers should be preventable. While eating fibre in fruit, vegetables and porridge has not been proven to prevent bowel cancer it can have beneficial effects on the bowel, body weight and on blood cholesterol. Screening for bowel cancer by a combination of faecal specimen testing for blood, and bowel examination, especially in those with a family history of bowel cancer, can save a lot of lives. Soon non-invasive bowel imaging may be available.

While disease prevention must remain a major goal, it is important that consideration be given to those in outlying areas with health problems such as cancer and heart disease. If cancer treatment is only available at major medical centres, the HSE policy of 'equality for all' will have to ensure that overnight accommodation in the centre is available to patients and relatives. This would go a long way to alleviate the stress from illness, travel and emotional upset. The use of invasive procedures for patients with life-threatening heart conditions does not necessarily improve survival. In the UK, patients admitted to highly specialised hospitals had a poorer outcome than those equally-ill patients treated in local units. The risk of major bleeding and stroke was also higher in people with acute heart problems who were treated in specialist hospitals. This argues against the early routine transfer of patients with a cardiac condition to hospitals with highly specialised facilities, and for a more selective use of invasive procedures. However, it is essential that local units be equipped to deal appropriately with the situation, for example a heart attack must be treated according to a standard accepted state-of-the-art protocol. It would also be good policy and appropriate resources made available for this, if an audiovisual link could be established between the 'expert' centre and other locations.

RTA figures for the Republic of Ireland are one of the highest in the EU and this situation has remained unchanged for many years. Ireland does not enforce its traffic laws particularly with regard to speeding and drink-driving. Drivers in Ireland include a significant number of young men who race everywhere and impatient middle-aged men who drive fast cars with little or no regard for speed limits. Road rage seems to be increasing. In our cities, pedestrians have no respect for traffic lights. In the first 240 days of 2005 there have been 244 deaths on the road, essentially one needless death per day. Every weekend there are usually at least three deaths from RTAs involving mainly young men, and car crashes are one of the leading causes of deaths in adolescents who drive with excessive speed on roads not designed for high-powered cars. The contribution to RTAs from excess alcohol intake is substantial. Cocaine intake and lack of sleep may also be contributory. Suicidal ideation in young drivers may well be a further cause.

Poor reading ability and colour blindness (affecting males) may be contributory to the road accident rate. Dyslexia is said to affect the way in which the brain processes sensory information and this can have a negative impact on co-ordination and a driver's reactions. Dyslexia may therefore be a factor in RTAs. Damage to an area of the brain called the angular gyrus affects the written word and may be responsible for some cases of dyslexia. There is some recent controversy however, over whether or not dyslexia is actually a disease entity. It has been postulated that the condition may not be due to brain damage but may arise because subjects have not been adequately taught how to read. Parents and primary school teachers must be able to at least recognise that a child's performance is not adequate and refer for evaluation for dyslexia. Dyslexic subjects are often high achievers so parents must ensure that their child is appropriately evaluated. No child should be allowed to leave school illiterate or semi-literate.

Sleep apnoea, a condition affecting spontaneous breathing, occurs mainly in obese individuals and makes subjects almost 10-times more likely to have an RTA.

The contribution of ADHD to RTAs in Ireland is not available but may be significant. All accidents may be higher in people with ADHD. Impulsive conduct can lead to school problems. If not diagnosed and treated, the ADHD subject will become uneducated and may be involved in a variety of anti-social behaviour such as theft and arson, cruelty to animals and people. ADHD can be caused by excess alcohol intake during pregnancy. There are no medical tests for ADHD however a safe diagnosis must be made to avoid incorrect child 'labelling'. ADHD can be treated with psychotherapy, appropriate education, family involvement and medication.

RTAs are lower on dual carriageways. There is paucity of dual carriageways in Ireland and on some of the existing motorways there is lack of capacity. Most accidents occur on narrow roads. The use of a stone mastic asphalt on road surfaces instead of asphalt may reduce noise but may have a poorer grip. Most accidents are however caused by human error. What can be done about human error ?

Speed cameras may not make the roads safer and there is some evidence that they just shift accidents further up the road. However they do have a role in targeting the persistently-offending driver. More crash barriers and anti-skid surfaces on the roads, increased numbers of crossings and better monitoring of speed limits on narrow country roads would decrease accidents. Gardaí must be strategically placed on single carriageway and narrow roads to allow apprehension of road abusers and an anarchic legal system that allows offenders to get away with trivial and inappropriate technicalities must be replaced. Driving tests must be updated and there must be a better throughput. Reform of the regulations governing motorbike riding and training is urgently needed with particular attention to law enforcement prohibiting drivers with provisional licences from carrying pillion passengers. Drivers with provisional licences must not be allowed to drive unaccompanied, under any circumstance. Breathalysers replace the need to take a blood or urine sample for alcohol testing. These tests must be robust and properly used in order to avoid any possible legal equivocation about the result. Gardaí must be instructed in how to use both roadside and garda station breathalysers. Random testing for drugs other than alcohol must also be introduced. Drivers who break the law by driving under the influence of alcohol or drugs or by speeding, must be penalised by a high monetary fine and have their licences removed for a time commensurate with the offence. The presence of a garda as an observer at busy traffic lights at peak traffic hours in cities is always a reassuring sign and might deter pedestrians from jay walking, and drivers from rushing through a red light. In the UK a system which fines and sends speeding or poor drivers back to driving school is used in certain regions. A similar system is necessary in Ireland where the road accident rate per population is much higher than in the UK. The UK has a much better drink-driving and speeding enforcement than Ireland.

In spite of the large numbers of head injuries relative to our population, major injuries which occur every weekend cannot be realistically treated in small local A&E departments. With the suggested reforms of the Irish Health Services it is likely that the percentage of the population reaching an adequately resourced A & E department within one hour following a road traffic accident would actually fall by approximately 10%. Treatment within one hour is vital as the 'golden hour' is the period when treatment is likely to produce the best outcome. An expert review of the reforms has suggested that relocation of ambulance services might be necessary, with ambulances being based at designated locations in communities rather than at ambulance bases. In response to this suggestion there are now plans for rapid response ambulance services for the Mid-West. The proposed Health Service reforms will need review particularly given our huge RTA rate, but accident prevention or at least reduction must remain the major goal.

There is no reason to think that subjects with epilepsy, high blood pressure, cardiac problems or diabetic patients taking insulin, make a substantial contribution to RTAs however as with all road users, subjects taking tablets or injections must be conversant with the medical aspects of fitness to drive for their own sake and for public safety. It is important to be stabilized on tablets or injections before driving. It is also important to be aware of what must be declared regarding eyesight and health when applying for a driving licence. This information is available at vehicle licensing centres.

Many teenagers have experimented with drugs. Heroin abuse has been particularly prevalent in 15-24year-old males, causing a drifting away from school at an early age, thus starting a downward spiral of addiction with little or no education and no lifetime skills. 50- 70% of prison admissions have been the result of crime committed in order to fund drug addiction and it is disturbing that 25% of offenders in some prisons may be former psychiatric patients. Perhaps if the psychiatric complaint was addressed the drug problem might not have arisen. The Merchants Quay Ireland 2003 Report shows that the numbers of drug users attending the Health Promotion Unit increased by up to 5% in 2003. Although government figures in early 2004 suggested that heroin use had decreased this may not be the case, and there is an increase in the use of cocaine. Unfortunately, once the brain circuits for addiction are established, the motivational effects of drugs are as strong as the desire for food or sex. Therefore measures must be in place to tackle the supply and demand for illicit drugs and prevention programmes in schools and in the workplace must remain the primary focus. Prevention is always better and easier than cure.

Education and life skills must be the basis for progress. School and community prevention programmes encouraging young people to live healthy lifestyles have begun to show some results with improvement in school attendance. The disruptive or unwilling pupil is often that way because of poor home conditions, lack of understanding of the subject being taught or poor stimulation by the environment into which he feels he is pushed. He may be emotionally unprepared for school and tends to behave like a younger pupil. Nurture with more time being given to him at school, home support plus zero tolerance may be the key to better discipline at home and at school. Adequate discipline must be started and continued from nursery through infant school to primary education. Recreational drugs must be avoided. Parents and teachers must emphasise that drug expectations always exceed reality and that an initial thrill is replaced, by a lifetime of misery and illness, or death. While all cases of illicit drug taking, alcoholism, suicide and sexual promiscuity will not be eliminated, education with primary prevention programmes in schools will at least give an insight into the perils of these activities and will lead to their reduction.

The fact that premature death and disability are caused by the use of mood-altering drugs or alcohol abuse before the age of 50 years, must be continually emphasized. Support programmes for children of drug users and one-parent families have been initiated. To prevent further drug addiction and alcoholism, other causes of homelessness such as poverty, housing shortages, the high cost of rented accommodation, relationship breakdown or mental health problems, all need to be addressed. While emergency shelters are necessary, these must be kept to a minimum and state and voluntary organizations should place greater emphasis on provision of long-term housing solutions. Subjects with problems have responsibility too and need to avail of services to help them stop abusing themselves, their families and their surroundings. The best treatment for homelessness is to address any mental health issues and to help with employment. Every support must be given to allow a homeless person to get either supervised or other suitable employment.

Many medicines available without prescription have the potential for misuse. People have to act responsibly and use these medicines only on a short-term basis. Education can help people to understand the dangers of alcohol and drugs, however every individual particularly those with a family history of any form of addiction, must use that knowledge to protect themselves, their family and their neighbours from substance abuse.

Parents too need support. Sleep disorders resulting from the pressures of modern life may cause a considerable proportion of relationships to break up. The demands of juggling a career, family and social life may sometimes prove exhausting. The pressure to conform and status anxiety are part of society in Ireland. Irritability, excessive smoking or drinking, inability to concentrate or to sleep can cause work or family disruption. To avoid stress causing serious physical ailments an appraisal of what you can and cannot do must be made. Tasks must be delegated and shared with the family. Avoid smoking, smokers and too much sun, eat sensibly, avoid alcohol excess and binge drinking and exercise as much as possible. A sensible approach to relaxation, family enjoyment, getting fitter and healthier is the wise course. Music can be very relaxing. Cut back on stimulants like coffee and tea. Exercise several hours before bedtime. Try to avoid using sleeping pills. Some recent research has indicated that in middle-aged men sleep disturbance is associated with increased risk of developing diabetes. This may be linked with the fact that sleep deprivation causes people to eat excessively thereby risking becoming obese. A good bed is a great investment! Heated water beds and electric blankets may not be ideal and should be used wisely if you want to start a family since the increased temperature may decrease fertility in males.

Parents need to guide their children by example- by not smoking, moderate alcohol, avoidance of recreational and non-prescription drugs, maintenance of moderate weight and exercising as much as possible. Mental stimulation of children must be made a priority by healthy nutrition and school attendance.

The problems in the Health Service will not be solved by extra funding. The nature of the health service in any country means that there are finite rather than infinite funds and there will never be an ideal situation where beds can be found instantly for every subject. Solutions will only be found by appropriate use of resources. This means good medicine, good management but decreased bureaucracy, proper use of hospital beds with timely discharges and appropriate use of long-term and convalescent facilities. Sometimes extra beds will have to be fitted into wards but that should not be a major problem with the necessary resourcefulness and pragmatism. In the case of mental health it appears that there may have been a huge drop in bed numbers over the past twenty years while at the same time there has not been an adequate compensatory increase in community support. Approximately 40% of homeless people in Ireland are said to have mental problems. If this is indeed the case then at least 2000 beds should now be provided in sheltered accommodation while all homeless individuals should at least have access to an adequately regulated hostel bed. Re-housing for the homeless must become feasible with better deployment of already available funds, however the homeless must put some effort into their own rehabilitation. It remains to be seen if the new hierarchy in the health system can promote the laudable aspirations of equality, fairness, patient-centred and accountability, however prevention of illness and reduction of alcohol consumption must be the main goal.

Key sentence: Prevention of illness and reduction of alcohol consumption must be the main goal.

2

Education

Education has a huge role in meeting the vast amount of social, cultural, political and health requirements of society. Education from an early age is essential to promote exercise, good eating habits, absence of smoking, moderation in alcohol intake, avoidance of drugs and care of the environment. Education about avoiding cruelty to animals must also be given at home and in schools. Children who abuse animals may also abuse people. Education must also play a role in decreasing Ireland's shamefully high road death rate. Ireland has one of the highest illiteracy rates in the European Union with 25% of the age group 16-64 years at the lowest level of literacy. Thirty percent of students in underprivileged areas suffer from severe literacy problems. Being able to read affects confidence and behaviour. Poor communication is a barrier to health and there is a significant correlation between low literacy rates and poor health. It would appear that child development is now no longer addressed in the home, in the school or in the wider society context.

Adults and children regardless of age must be encouraged if at all possible to learn to read, because this is vital for life-long confidence and well-being. All children with disabilities must be given education to suit their level of ability. ADHD subjects must be given appropriate attention to find their niche and divert them away from anti-social behaviour. Appropriate teaching and proper parenting must have major roles in the treatment of all children. If properly taught, most children of average intelligence can become high achievers. Resources must be concentrated on giving excellent education rather than on social handouts which may not benefit the child at all.

The signs of illiteracy must be recognised in order for help to be given. All persons who have difficulty communicating should in the appropriate setting be asked about their reading and writing skills. Relatives of subjects who cannot read or write must assist such people to overcome this disability by declaring it, doing something about it and overcoming it. Work place literacy programmes and family-based initiatives must be encouraged by every means possible. In the UK, a teacher has claimed that she can teach virtually any child to read. She concentrates on teaching the sounds of letters and helps children combine these to make words. Her methods are based on 'synthetic phonics' which means a way of building up words from basic sounds. This is not altogether new and in the past has been used with other methods. Using this system alone, children learn 44 pure letter sounds from pictures. Gradually their vocabulary increases and reading can be achieved in a remarkably short period of time. Parents can do this programme at home with their children and obviously illiterate adults can learn too. While learning, the brain is challenged. The phrase 'Use it or lose it' is particularly applicable to the brain. A mind challenged by reading is likely to remain alert while an unchallenged brain stops learning and may deteriorate.

The high illiteracy rate may be explained by a persistently elevated school drop-out rate. In Ireland overall, 81 % of students, stay on to Leaving Certificate. In the poorer areas, many second-level schools have dropout rates of 50% or more before taking Leaving Cert. More than 3000 subjects leave the system every year without any qualifications and boys are much more likely to leave school prematurely than girls. Less than 10% of traveller children obtain their Leaving Cert. Despite the current job choice many people lack employable skills and find it difficult to get suitable work.

93% of primary school children miss at least 12 days of school per year, 26% of second-level students in poorer areas miss school for at least 20 days per year while 91% of all second level pupils miss 15 days or more. Some children may be leaving school semi-literate and without the same social skills as their peers because they stay or are kept away from school to look after drug- or alcohol-addicted parents. A strategy for the care of addicted parents, elderly parents or disabled relatives should be put in place and if necessary parents may have to be prosecuted for 'deficiency of education' cruelty to children. Parents must not, if possible, take holidays in term-time which disrupts school attendance.

One in 4 male school–leavers is becoming an apprentice in a trade. More than half of those going into apprenticeships have their Leaving Certificate which will allow them, once the boom in the construction industry is over, to resume education if desired. For those who do not have any formal education the lure of money now may be a temptation to leave school early and semi-literate. It is important to be aware that courses are available to supply such people with guidance and training to prevent them being left behind in a knowledge economy. Immigrants are often more knowledgeable than the domestic population, particularly the unskilled domestic population. Up to 30% of the Irish workforce is low-skilled so the time to take action must be in childhood. In all primary schools the value of education must be emphasised to all strata of society particularly those living in poorer areas. Schemes have also commenced to tackle unemployment among people with disabilities. This is necessary to ensure total social inclusion, self-esteem and well-being.

No children should be made to feel failures if a more imaginative educational system is forthcoming to enable all to have a niche in society. Handouts without structured education are of little benefit to socially-deprived people often living in areas of vandalism and crime. Early education, extra teachers and parental support and guidance must be emphasised. All parents must take responsibility for educating themselves and their children. The message must be "No education, no future. Return to parents' low socio-economic status with repeat of cycle of educational poverty". All young children must be urged to stay in education for as long as possible. Everyone needs to learn as much as possible. The only way to do this is to ask the right questions and to make the right decisions. If one subject is boring then an alternative can be found. Parents must insist that their child can at least read, write and do basic maths with or without a calculator, before leaving primary school. If they cannot do this, the child will be condemned to a twilight existence for life as learning to read later on in life is that much more difficult but of course not impossible.

For an adult who has little or no ability to read, the temptation to say "It is too late to begin" must be resisted. The habit of falling asleep in front of the television after the evening meal does not indicate stupidity or lack of willpower but a lack of energy, being stuck in a rut and a need for a mental and physical makeover. The TV remote control must therefore be regularly set aside in order to attend the nearest literacy classes available, to take a walk with or without the dog and to get a new hobby. However, that does not mean that one should never watch TV. Watching a favourite sitcom or listening to music are great stress-busters so indulge from time to time but not all of the time! The absolute priority must be to learn to read, write and count money and by so doing, to develop alternative interests to alcohol and television!

Unruly children are often sidelined at school. It is essential to investigate the cause of the bad behaviour because there is usually a reason for this. The subject is often male and may come from a family with social problems. He may have undiagnosed ADHD or is just badly-behaved and has had poor parenting. Provisions for follow-up of such children must be made to ensure that they get adequate counselling and appropriate education. Schools that accept only the brightest pupils can often score highly in exams. Schools which accept students of varied ability often are criticized for getting lower grades. This is unfortunate because these schools often serve the community well and often manage to help the less-able students. These schools should be given extra resources to educate so-called 'problem' children. It is important to remember that the brightest child is often not the brightest adult and that 'problem' children are often the product of bad parenting and poor teaching. Not only do the poorer children lack education but a considerable number of people in the country, both rich and poor, lack social awareness with little civic spirit. In general, knowledge on basic scientific issues is below the European average. This must be addressed by a more innovative practical approach to the school curriculum. Better education will in time enable a better self security and sophistication. Traveller parents must ensure that their children attain good basic education in literacy and numeracy and go on to obtain either practical skills or further academic education at third level. To be educated is not snobbish or 'queer'. It is an essential part of life.

Mental illness amongst North County Dublin secondary school students is said to be high with 15% apparently having a psychiatric disorder. This is worrying and needs full investigation as to the underlying reasons. Children must have good nutrition. Physically-fit children do better in the classroom as well as in the playground. It is important to remember that what students eat and drink in the run-up to exams can significantly affect their performance. Parents must be supportive at exam time. Alcohol should not be allowed at any time during the formative years. Teenage abstinence is strongly influenced by a family environment where drinking is prohibited by parents.

Before leaving school all students must be fully informed regarding the rules of the road and the rights and duties of pedestrians, cyclists and motorists. Since Irish teenagers are losing their virginity earlier than ever with 10% of youths having sex by age 15 years, it is essential that information and the facts regarding the legal implications of early sex and age of consent, be at least mentioned in school. Studies from the UK and Mexico indicate that teaching 'safe sex' achieves little apart from a rise in promiscuity. Postponement of sexual experience with all its implications, until a later age, may perhaps be a more realistic aim.

Credit unions have begun a campaign to expand its network among schools. This is important as a means of teaching young people the value of money and of saving. It makes young people aware of how much things cost and how hard one needs to save to get both necessities and luxuries.

The National Adult Literacy Agency has recently declared that workers who did not study beyond the Junior Certificate should be given paid leave to improve their literacy and numeracy. This may be a good idea. All measures to improve literacy and numeracy in adults and children must be considered for the health and well-being of all of our citizens, however methods should be in place to avoid abuse of the system. A radical funding change with greater equality is needed in third-level education.

Key sentence: All young children must be urged to stay in education for as long as possible.

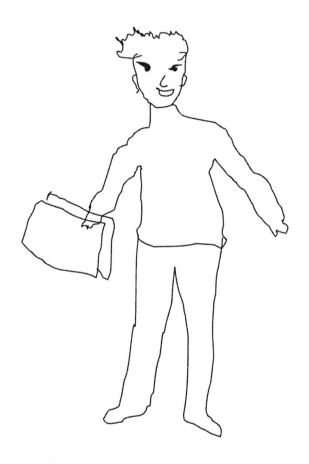

**I MUST LEARN HOW TO READ, WRITE AND COUNT
MONEY OR I WILL BE CALLED AN ILLITERATE PERSON**

3

Lifestyle

A high-risk lifestyle is defined as one where a person does not exercise, drinks excessive alcohol, smokes, and eats food high in 'bad' fats, high in salt, high in sugar and low in fibre. Too much stress and inadequate sleep can also contribute to a high-risk lifestyle. Stress is a big cause of absence from work, replacing back pain as the most commonly cited problem on medical certificates. 'Sick building syndrome' is said to be more related to stress than to an unhealthy building structure. Although young adults today have more money than any previous generation, they seem to be stressed and unhealthy with low levels of exercise, increasing levels of obesity, binge drinking, drug taking and depression. Smoking has increased significantly amongst Irish women making them more vulnerable to early heart disease. The prevalence of asthma has increased. Breast feeding has decreased. Lifestyle has decreased fertility in both men and women. Stress may lead to heart disease, stroke and diabetes because a cluster of risk factors called the 'metabolic syndrome' may follow from unhealthy lifestyle.

In recent years with unlimited resources in many countries including Ireland, 'excess' has become acceptable and expected. A combination of excess eating of processed foods with high salt intake while also drinking excess alcohol has led to obesity. It is recommended that males consume no more than 21 units of alcohol per week or 3 units per day and females no more than 14 units or 2 per day. A unit is a half pint of beer or 1 small glass of wine or a small measure of spirits. Alcopops each contain between 1 and 2 units. Excess alcohol leads to high blood pressure. Processed food means that a lot of essential fibre and vitamins have been removed. Stress and haste in swallowing large amounts too quickly has lead to hurried meals, bloated bodies, pot bellies and heartburn. 'Pot belly' means that too much weight is carried on the stomach and the body appearance looks like an apple. Diabetic patients who have an increased risk of heart disease often accumulate fat on the abdomen in this way. Even though an apple a day probably does keep the doctor away, an apple-shaped body is unhealthy with excess fat on the abdomen being positively linked with diabetes and heart disease. On the other hand a pear-shaped body with excess weight on the buttocks although not a beautiful sight is indeed healthier! Whatever your size do not wear tight waistbands or tight shirt collars since these may make you feel unwell by causing indigestion or dizzy symptoms respectively.

Recent research has also indicated that low fruit and vegetable consumption, the intake of sweetened drinks and excessive salt and alcohol are associated with an increased risk of high blood pressure, fat accumulation on the abdomen and an increased risk of diabetes. Subjects with high blood pressure, obesity, diabetes, heart disease or problems with the circulation perhaps due to smoking, are at an increased risk of stroke. Irish women are more likely to die from heart disease or stroke than from breast cancer. Stroke may cause paralysis or lack of coordination, disturbance of vision, swallowing, coughing or speech and is a common cause of death. Stroke follows a blood clot or blockage in the brain blood vessels or may follow a brain haemorrhage. Prevention is essential. Subjects with a family history of stroke should discuss this with their GP.

In Ireland poultry was once an excellent product. The hens and turkeys were allowed to have a life and people ate small adequate portions of nutritious meat. Now, here as in the UK, the 'battery bird' with excess fat seems to be the stable diet of people who seem unaware of the vast amounts of salt, fat and poor nutritional value of the processed poultry 'food' they are consuming on a daily basis. Healthy food choices keep you fit and strong and may prevent disease. Excess or unhealthy foods have the opposite effect. Meals must be eaten regularly, avoiding too many unhealthy snacks such as biscuits. Food must be enjoyed rather than taken into the mouth in vast quantities and regular exercise should be commenced. Regular moderate-intensity physical activity such as walking gives substantial health benefits. Try not to eat late at night in order to avoid digestion problems. Drinking alcohol with food shortly before bed-time can cause relaxation of the sphincter that keeps the food and digestive acids in the stomach, leading to 'heartburn'. Poor eating habits may lead to gullet and stomach problems.

Do not dwell too much on calories or weights. Be flexible but not extravagant and go easy on fattening poor-health promoting items like fizzy drinks. Replace salt on alternate days with pepper and or herbs. For those interested in calories (measured as kilocalories) women need approximately 2,000 and men 2500 kilocalories per day. Bad fats are saturated fats from animal sources and 'trans' fats. Butter is a saturated fat and although it tastes great it should be eaten in small to moderate amounts. 'Trans' or hydrogenated fats are margarines which are made solid by pumping hydrogen through oils and should be used in small amounts. 'Trans' fats may also be present in vegetable oils so all oils should be used in small amounts. Cook a meal containing vegetables and eat some fruit every day. Boiling, steaming or grilling are healthier ways of cooking than frying. Avoid fast-food on a regular basis. The excess fat in 'fast food' often includes over-used oils and salt which are not good for your health.

Most people who are overweight feel their clothes getting tighter however, before bursting the seams it is a good idea to have some measure of size. Body mass index (BMI) is an indicator of obesity. It has a disadvantage in that it does not specify where the excess weight is and excess weight on the abdomen as stated above is much more likely to cause diabetes and heart disease than excess weight on the buttocks. To find out your BMI divide your weight in kilograms by height in metres squared for example an 80kg man of height 1.8 metre has a BMI of 80 divided by (1.8 x1.8) 3.2 = 25 . BMI should be between 19 and 25 with values above 30 indicating obesity, and values over 40 indicating extreme obesity. A female waistline should be no greater than 88cm (35 inches) and preferably less (24-28 inches) while a male waistline should be no greater than 102cm (40 inches) and preferably less (28-34). To measure waist size, after breathing out use a suitably relaxed tape-measure at the mid-point between the rib margin and the hip margin.

- *1 pound = 0.45 kilogram,; 1 pound = 16oz and 1oz= 28 gram*

- *1 foot =0.3 metre ; 1 metre = 100cm and 1 inch = 2.54cm*

Many surveys have indicated that at mealtimes the number one choice for children are burgers, chips or pizzas. In fact as a consequence of eating fast food UK surveys have shown that many children can no longer use a knife and fork since most eating is done out of a container and there are few family meals. Teachers are obliged to train children in how to use a knife and fork because they are not learning basic social skills in the home! There is a lot of criticism of food companies who are said to target young children by advertising 'fast food' and 'soft drinks'. However, young people considered sufficiently mature to be given pocket money to buy food snacks also need to be informed of the recommended daily intake of fat (70 gram per day for women and 90 for men), salt (3-5 gram per day) and sugar (50-70 gram). Remember that food already contains some salt and natural sugar such as fructose from fruit and lactose from milk so the extra salt sprinkled on food and the teaspoons of sugar called sucrose added to food or drink should be kept to a minimum. Generally about 4 teaspoons per day of added sugar (sucrose, glucose syrup or maltose) are acceptable.

Catering companies would rather serve fast food which sells well rather than taking a risk with more healthy options which may not be as popular, because parents in general, have not trained their children to seek healthy options. Food served by take-aways and cafeterias are often rich in fat, salt and carbohydrate and usually there is no label to inform the eater regarding the amount of salt, fat and sugar being consumed. Frequent 'eating out' tends to lead to weight gain so home cooking should be a regular rather than an infrequent occurrence. Children enjoy 'fast foods' so their elimination is not realistic. However it is possible to limit the amount and frequency of consumption. Parents must understand that unlimited amounts of these foods may cause children of the twenty-first century to die before their parents so fast food once a week must be a treat and not a right. A practical approach in take-aways should be to use healthier cooking methods to cook the 'fast food', and to reduce the portions. Removing visible fat from meat before cooking and replacing high-fat gravy with a low-fat version would be a start. Boiling, stewing, grilling or steaming are low-fat cooking methods. In school cafeterias attractive healthy alternatives with steamed or boiled potato, pasta, meat or fish, vegetable and fruit should be made available alongside once weekly burger and chips and children encouraged from an early age to eat these. Habits form early and easily and Finnish children have been encouraged with great success, to adhere for the most part to a sensible healthy school lunch.

From an early age it is essential to reinforce the message that fresh fruit and vegetables are essential for a healthy diet. Fish should replace meat on a regular basis. Porridge is an excellent food which may prevent children from becoming overweight. This may be due to the fact that eating porridge prolongs energy levels and prevents snacking. Porridge oats also contain a type of fibre called beta-glycan which helps reduce cholesterol. Sugar-coated cereals should not be used frequently. Fizzy drinks should be restricted to once weekly. Essentially each of these is a drink of liquid sugar and the equivalent of several lollipops. Each fizzy drink may contain almost 4 teaspoons of sugar, which is the total allowance of added sugar per day. Added sugar includes sucrose or table sugar, glucose/glucose syrup, maltose and honey. Full fat milk is a good food or drink for children.

Most supermarket foods are labelled and most food companies' attitude is that it is up to the consumer to make an informed decision as to what he will eat. While this is a valid statement the company must take responsibility for adding unnecessary excessive amounts of salt, fat and sugar to make snacks more appetizing. Irish soup and sauce manufacturers have promised to reduce the amount of salt in their products by 10% and in some cases this may have already occurred. All food companies should be responsible for their advertisements and full information regarding their product should be given. The label should state the ingredients and whether or not any of these have been genetically modified (GM). TV advertising should reinforce the message that "For healthy living, eat and drink in moderation, vary your diet and take daily exercise ". Supermarkets should avoid price promotions on high calorie fatty foods or on hydrogenated fat-containing products such as biscuits. Sweets should not be displayed near the checkout. Fresh fruit of all sorts should instead be placed at children's eye level. Parents should undertake to give only sufficient pocket money to allow 'fast food' consumption once weekly.

Unless you are following a special diet for medical reasons there is no need to weigh your food however it is good to know about portion size. Buying low calorie food is expensive and unnecessary since it is much wiser to eat normal food in moderate sensible amounts.

A serving for one person is about 100 gram
low calorie means equal to or less than 40 kcals
lean is less than 10 gram of fat, less than 4 gram of saturated fat and less than 0.1 gram of cholesterol per 100 gram serving

20 gram of fat or more per 100 gram of food is a lot
3 gram of fat or less per 100 gram of food is a little
1 gram of saturated fat or less per 100 gram of food is a small amount
low cholesterol is less than 0 .05 gram of cholesterol per 100 gram serving

10 gram sugar or more per 100 gram of food is a lot
2 gram or less sugar per 100 gram of food is a little

3 gram of fibre per 100 gram of food is a lot
0.5 gram of fibre per 100 gram of food is a little
1 pound = 16oz, ;1o z =28 gram
1 gram = 1000mg
1 pint = 550ml approx

Daily intake of salt (which is sodium chloride), should be up to 5 gram per day, depending on the size of person. To translate from sodium to salt multiply by 2.5.
Special diets require low intake of salt:
low-sodium means less than 0.10 gram of sodium or 0.25 gram of salt per 100 gram serving

very low sodium is less than .04 gram of sodium or 0.1 gram of salt per 100 gram serving.

The food label should state the weight in the container, the amount of calories, the protein, fat and carbohydrate contents. The salt content will usually be listed. The fats will be given as saturated, polyunsaturated or monosaturated. Saturated are animal fats, polyunsaturated are fish and vegetable oils and monosaturated are olive and nut oils. The label should tell you if the product contains 'a little' or 'a lot' of sugar, fat, salt or fibre.

An innovative pilot project at an Irish school indicates that children can learn to behave very sensibly. A typical lunch at that school now includes a piece of fruit, a sandwich and milk. Allowed foods include protein-rich ones such as meat, eggs and tinned fish, fruit including apples, bananas, mandarins and tasty vegetables such as cucumber and carrots. Drinks include milk, water, unsweetened fruit juice and yoghurt drinks. Not allowed are crisps, peanuts, chewing gum, lollipops and fizzy drinks. Some sweets are allowed on one day per week. Re-use of containers is advised to cut down on litter. Plastic wrapping is kept to a minimum. This is a great start and already has been copied in other schools. It should be copied nationwide. While full-calorie fizzy and soft drinks should not be consumed on a regular basis, like all dietary substances these can if desired be taken on rare occasions. It is also important for parents to be supportive of sensible nutritious food for their children. In the UK, support for healthy school dinners has taken some time to become established but gradually parents are being won over and rather than supplying fizzy drinks and crisps, they are actively encouraging their children to eat the dinners.

It is important to be aware of a few small steps which can make your diet instantly more healthy. While cooking have good ventilation so open a window if possible! Oven-frying using a crumb coating leaves foods relatively fat-free. Stir-frying uses very little fat and flavour is retained with crisp vegetables. Do not however overheat the oil or the non-stick coating. Skim fat from gravy before serving, using a gravy separator. Do not heap food onto the plate. Eat moderate portions and do not have second helpings. Use all fats in small amounts. It is essential to eat as slowly as possible. Eating quickly causes too much food to be eaten too quickly and can cause indigestion with heartburn. Cancer of the oesophagus or gullet is increasing in all developed countries often from years of heartburn with reflux of acid into the gullet, however it may also be caused by elimination of essential micro-organisms from the stomach by excessive or inappropriate use of antibiotics. Once essential micro-flora are interfered with, nature often rebels and causes disease. It is essential not to restrict any foods completely unless a medical condition requires this, because long-term restriction only invites 'blow-outs' when food is consumed so excessively as to nullify weeks or months of restriction. Modify the diet rather than restrict completely.

Too much salt or alcohol increase blood pressure with risk of stroke. Processed foods such as pizza, cornflakes, sausages, white bread and instant 'teledinners' contain excessive salt. To avoid excess salt intake these foods should be taken occasionally rather than frequently, no extra salt should be scattered on the food and salt should from time to time be substituted with pepper, herbs or spices in moderate amounts. Soya sauce is nice and also nutritious but should not be used excessively because it contains a fairly large amount of salt. Chips may taste good but look at them when cold- they are often greasy and should be avoided or taken infrequently. In addition the chips may contain acrylamide, a chemical produced in some foods which are prepared at high temperatures.

Most people think that salads are a healthy option which they should be, however be wary of what is added to the salad. Avoid or take little mayonnaise. Dressings should be vinaigrette- or tomato-based, avoiding excessive sugar or fat although of course richer dressings can be eaten on occasions! Try to choose from lean meat or organic poultry, fish, eggs, beans of all varieties, boiled or baked potatoes, rice, pasta, wholegrain bread, fresh fruit and lightly boiled vegetables. Use average portions and do not have 'seconds'. Porridge is great for breakfast however some people prefer bread. Have a couple of slices of bread if you wish for breakfast. Avoid the Irish custom of having 2 slices of bread and butter in addition to the evening meal of potatoes or rice, vegetable and meat or fish. Manual workers in the construction industry use up a lot of calories and may feel that they need bread in addition to the evening meal . This is reasonable provided they do not become too fat by eating excessive take-aways and drinking excessive alcohol. Binge drinking is presently a big problem in the building industry. This may be due to stress and must be addressed by reducing the ongoing pressure to reach deadlines.

Use unsweetened juice or low-calorie drinks but the latter should not be used excessively. Low-calorie drinks contain artificial sweeteners which appear to be safe however they may perpetuate a need for sweet drinks. Recently researchers in Italy have raised some health concerns about aspartame, the artificial sweetener which is used in many food and drink products. Further studies are ongoing. Aspartame should not be used in subjects with a medical condition called phenylketonuria. (PKU). One teaspoonful of sugar is acceptable over porridge or in hot drinks but avoid excessive sugar in tea or coffee. It is wise to avoid using tinned foods every day by using fresh vegetables, fish and lean meat when possible.

Drink some water with mid-day and evening meals. If you drink alcohol, drink sensibly and preferably with meals. When drinking alcohol, alternate with water or diet fizzy drinks. Avoid low-carbohydrate alcoholic drinks because these have a high alcohol content. **Never drink and drive** since even a small amount of alcohol can affect the driving ability in certain individuals and this effect may not be predictable.

Remember the saying 'Breakfast like a king, lunch like a prince and have an evening meal like a pauper'? The rationale here is to eat well at breakfast time in order to work with energy while avoiding mid-morning snacks, and eat less before going to bed as the calories may not be worked off and may cause indigestion. While of course you do not need to get fanatical about taking excesses occasionally, do not get into a habit of doing so. An extra chocolate biscuit every day may make you fat over a period of 12 months. For a mid-morning or mid-afternoon snack have a piece of fresh fruit with a suitable non-alcoholic drink. Avoid regular sugary drinks. Dried fruits such as apricots or raisins in small amounts are useful snacks but pay attention to the teeth by brushing or drinking some water. Since dried fruit can contain a lot of glucose syrup or sucrose it is wise not to eat more than a few pieces at once. Use the packet over a series of snacks but alternate with fresh fruit.

What is the practical way to achieve a balance? Avoid big portions. Use all fats and oils in small amounts. For the Lotharios amongst us remember that less fat apparently leads to better sexual prowess! Butter should be used in small amounts. Vegetable oil in small amounts can also be used a couple of times per week. Try to use olive oil, rapeseed or peanut oil in small amounts a couple of times per week. Peanut oil must be avoided if there is a history of nut allergy. Olive oil preparations, in addition to 'good' fats, may contain anti-inflammatory agents which are beneficial in preventing diseases like diabetes and fatty artery deposits. Fresh fruit and some vegetable consumption is important on a daily basis. Fruit can best be eaten between meals with due attention to teeth washing however sweet and sour combinations e.g. fruit with savoury is also very appetizing. A chopped raw apple (the skin must be washed but used, as a lot of vitamin C is contained in the skin), a piece of melon or grapes enhance any meal while making it healthy and the fibre content helps offset excess fat absorption. Starchy foods such as potato, bread, pasta or rice are important to replenish the glycogen stores in muscle. It can take up to 48 hours to replenish the glycogen. Protein from meat, fish, poultry, beans or eggs is important to build up tissue, and levels of serotonin and dopamine, substances important in nerve signal transmission.

Use bread (wholegrain or granary are good), cereal such as porridge or small amounts of muesli, potato, rice (brown is preferable as it contains more vitamins) and pasta, plain or fruit yoghurt, milk or low fat milk, small amounts of cheese or low fat cheese, beans, peas and lentils, moderate amounts of lean meat, poultry and fish as the backbone of your daily diet. Try to eat fish twice weekly as it contains the essential fatty acid omega-3. Omega-3 is also present in organic milk, spinach and nuts. Garlic bread can of course be eaten in moderation but avoid too much garlic butter! A few crackers and cheese can be eaten occasionally. Fruit yoghurt contains a significant amount of sugar so avoid adding sugar to tea to balance things up! Manufacturers should reduce the sugar content of yoghurts, these could still taste well with a lower amount of added sugar.

Confectionary, cakes, biscuits and snacks such as crisps should not be eaten regularly. These will add fat because of the fat and sugar content. The excess sugar carbohydrate gets converted into fat. Low-fat crisps have less fat than full-fat crisps but should be reserved for rare occasions. However tasty the following are, they must be used sparingly since each has a substantial percentage of ' bad 'fat (saturated or 'trans' fat present): butter, margarine, double or single cream, beef-burgers, cheese, sausages, biscuits, cakes, chocolates and bacon. Although butter contains saturated fat it does not have 'trans' fat while margarine contains 'trans ' fat and no saturated fat so small amounts of either are advised. If chocolate is eaten try and buy a good product as the higher the cocoa content the better it is for you! Remember that there is no need to eliminate these products entirely from the diet, just use in sensible low to moderate amounts. Ice-cream can be eaten in small to moderate amounts on occasions because its glycaemic index is relatively low, but do not eat it every day! To avoid infection always make sure that the ice-cream is solid and not runny.

Have as much variety as possible. If your funds are limited remember bread, potatoes, beans, tomatoes, fruit, portions of meat, fish and cheese are a lot cheaper and healthier than 'ready to go' meals. Do not skip main meals because you will then compensate by regularly eating bad snacks of biscuits, cheap sweets and chocolate, and fat-containing cakes. Good snacks include a glass of water, about 2 tablespoons of mixed nuts and raisins, about 10 grapes, 2 squares of chocolate (chocolate containing 60% cocoa is good), yoghurt, a piece or two of any fresh fruit and any portion of vegetables.

In the next chapter a more detailed explanation of why certain foods are recommended will be given and glycaemic index will also be discussed.

Once the diet is on track it is important to avoid excessive stress which can have negative effects on lifestyle. Stress in some form or another is a normal component of life, however in some individuals it can have devastating effects. The adverse effects of stress may occur in many different forms and produce illness of many varieties. Smoking or alcohol dependence cause body stress. Some other common stressors include work- or home-related events, driving, sex particularly with a new partner, lack or disturbance of sleep or reversal of sleep pattern in night workers, or being aware of 'illness in the family'. It is also important to be aware that symptoms of stress can be caused by excessive intake of caffeine in coffee, tea, fizzy drinks, some anti-pain tablets or nasal decongestants. The effects of stress may be particularly hazardous to the patient suffering from a heart disorder, to the older patient and to the female undergoing hormonal changes related to her reproductive functions. Exercise can reduce stress. Taking the dog for a walk can be stress-relieving provided he does not take you for a walk! Music is a stress reducer and can also have a beneficial effect on pain. It is important to stop smoking and to keep alcohol consumption at a healthy level or avoid completely if alcoholism runs in the family. It is important too, to get adequate sleep and if required, to get adequate advice with regard to work, marriage and hormonal adjustment. Smoking and watching television on a continuous basis are habits that can be changed with determination although your GP can help with the smoking addiction.

There is some evidence that sleep deprivation, perhaps as a result of a wild lifestyle may bring about hormonal changes that promote obesity. People who stay up late may also tend to smoke. In seasonal affective disorder (SAD), depression is blamed on lack of UV light. This condition increases the longer the winter nights and has a 1% incidence in Florida and a 10% incidence in Alaska. People with this condition eat a lot and have restless sleep with craving for extra sleep, suggesting a hibernation-like effect. The cure is to use simulated daylight by using bright lamps thus artificially lengthening the winter days.

Patients with heart disease should get sound cardiac advice before getting involved in recreations involving considerable physical stress. It is important to wear good warm clothes in winter and to avoid pushing the car in all weathers, particularly cold weather!

One of the main problems with ageing is increasing isolation from others in the community. To avoid this, the older person must be given every assistance to participate in society by attention to vision, hearing and by the use of walking aides.

An estimated 93% of Irish people suffer from some degree of gum disease. Gum disease is the main cause of tooth loss in adults. Any bleeding when brushing means gum disease and needs attention because your teeth may loosen and fall out. Gum disease can also increase the risk of heart disease from infection. Vitamin D, (it is formed in the skin from the effect of sunlight or can be taken in the diet for example in cheese or eggs), may help to reduce gum disease. While crowning and bridging may sometimes be required, these are costly and when performed for cosmetic reasons alone may replace a natural look with a rather artificial smile so do not crown unless it is necessary. Keep your teeth healthy by brushing after food or sweet drinks. Avoid vigorous brushing, this is unnecessary. Do not smoke as your breath will smell and gum disease is higher in smokers. See a dentist at least occasionally. Nowadays, apart from your pocket there is little pain and a lot of gain from a dental visit!

If you have your hair coloured make sure that you use a reputable colorant. Alopecia (loss of scalp hair) can be difficult to treat, so eat sensibly, try not to get stressed and avoid harsh hair treatments. If you want hair extensions do not use them indefinitely. Think twice about sun worship either by exposure to the sun or to sun beds. Some sun is necessary for all of us in order to strengthen our bones however excess sun exposure is unwise. 15 minutes sun exposure a day, avoiding the noon to 1400 hour period as the sun may be very hot during this time, is sufficient for vitamin D formation. Better be pale and interesting rather than have prematurely aged skin and the risk of skin cancer. Irish and Scottish people have very sensitive skin and are at high risk for skin cancer. Sun causes irreversible changes to the skin so if planning on sitting in the sun use appropriate sun-block and if necessary a hat. It is also wise to remember that sun-block against UVA and UVB rays is the best anti-ageing cream available, however it has to be used continuously as its effects are of limited duration. Sunscreen contains para-aminobenzoic acid (PABA) which may cause allergy in some individuals. A PABA-free waterproof sun lotion is now available.

Children and teenagers less than 18 years old should not be exposed to sun-beds. The long-term consequences are unknown.

Unlicensed skin-lightening creams must not be used.

For those who like to talk, be careful not to overuse mobile phones. There is no definite evidence that the emissions from mobile phones cause disease however further studies may need to be done. While listening or talking, alternate the phone between ears. It is also a good idea to alternate the site where the phone is carried. A hand-free kit is useful. Hand-held mobile phones should not be used while driving. These increase accident risk. Children should not use mobile phones on a regular basis since the risk of emissions having effects on the growing brain has not been adequately studied. The part of the brain involved in inhibiting risky behaviour (the prefrontal cortex) is not fully formed in a teenager and in some individuals may not mature fully until well over twenty years of age.

Radiation from mobile phones, computers and microwave ovens can all add up and could be causing headaches, joint pain, depression and fatigue so do not overuse these devices if possible. Avoid loud noise. Damage to the ear nerve may occur. Ear plugs may be necessary at concerts where it is wise to sit as far away from loudspeakers as possible.

Key sentences: A high-risk lifestyle is defined as one where a person does not exercise, drinks excessive alcohol, smokes, and eats food high in 'bad' fats, high in salt, high in sugar and low in fibre. From an early age it is essential to reinforce the message that daily fresh fruit and vegetables are essential for a healthy diet.

4

In The Kitchen

Eating the "right" food is the key to a healthier, fitter and a happier lifestyle. It is true that good health is our biggest wealth so it must be protected. Children and adults can increase their energy levels and their concentration by eating plenty of fruit and vegetables and avoiding too much sugar and too much fat.

Consumer concerns about the traceability of foods, the environment and animal welfare must be considered in the overall animal processing chain.

A healthy diet is one that is based around a content of:

- 10-15% protein

- 20-30% of fat: monosaturated (10-15%) from olive oil polyunsaturated (up to 10%) from fish and vegetable oil and saturated (less than 10%) fat from lean meat

- salt 3-5 gram per day

- 45-50% carbohydrate from starchy and sugary food including; potatoes, beans, pasta, rice, bread, milk (starchy) fruit and vegetables (containing fructose, vitamins, minerals and fibre)

- sugar per day of 50-70 gram. (This includes natural sugars and added sugar)

- at least 20 gram per day of fibre from fresh fruit, vegetables and porridge.

Carbohydrate is present in rice, potatoes, bread, beans and fruit. Sugars are present naturally in starchy food and in fruit. Added sugar includes table sugar which is sucrose, glucose/glucose syrup and invert syrup present for example in sweets, maltose in beer and honey. Dried fruit may also contain sucrose or glucose syrup. Obviously it is important to keep the added sugars to a minimum. All carbohydrates increase the blood sugar levels. The sugars will raise it quickly while the starchy foods will help to control it.

Low-calorie sweeteners can be a useful alternative to sugar, however like all foods they should not be used all the time but on occasions for example when a 'sweet binge' might lead to excessive sugar consumption.

Protein is provided from meat, poultry, fish, eggs, nuts and pulses such as beans, peas or lentils. Pulses also provide carbohydrate. Eggs provide high quality protein and supply more of the essential amino acids than any other protein. One egg contributes approximately 10% of the daily recommended protein. Although cholesterol is present in egg yolk, if eggs are eaten in moderation (not more than 4-6 per week) the blood cholesterol does not tend to rise. Egg yolk also contains a range of vitamins (vitamins A, B, D and E) and minerals such as iron, calcium, iodine, phosphate, zinc and selenium. Protein is needed at any age but particularly in childhood and adolescence, for tissue growth and regeneration. Daily protein requirement is approximately 3 oz. Too much meat protein is unnecessary and may increase the risk of gut cancer.

There are three types of fats in the food that we eat- saturated fat generally from meat sources, polyunsaturated fat from fish, nuts and vegetable cooking oil and monosaturated fat from olive and (pea) - nut oil. Blood cholesterol rises the more saturated fat intake increases however although meat contains saturated fat it also contains protein, vitamin B_{12}, iron and zinc so a moderate amount of lean meat can be included in the diet. Omega-3 and omega-6 are known as essential fatty acids and it is important for all of us to take them in small amounts. Oily fish such as salmon, tuna and mackerel contains omega-3. Organic milk also contains omega-3. The cows are given a special fish oil blend along with their normal feed. Omega-3 lowers blood fats and the stickiness of blood. 'Sticky' blood is not healthy as clots may form as a result of the stickiness. Omega-3 also blocks inflammatory substances in the blood which if present in large amounts can trigger heart disease or other inflammatory diseases such as arthritis. Eating fish once or twice a week is a good idea and may be beneficial for prevention of heart disease, diabetes and rheumatoid arthritis. Claims have also been made for improvements in ADHD and for improvement in cognitive problems in dyslexic children. Omega-6 fats are present in nut oil, meat, eggs and blended fat spreads such as margarine. Small amounts of oils or spreads are sufficient for essential fat replacement. It is wise to eat omega-3 and omega-6 foods roughly in similar proportions since excessive omega-6 may raise oestrogen levels but omega-3 tends to block the effect of excessive oestrogen and boosts immunity. Monosaturated fat from olive oil and polyunsaturated fat from vegetable oil should form part of the diet. Olive oil may prevent inflammation. *All oils and spreads should be consumed in small to moderate amounts as too much may cause weight gain.* Small to moderate means a coating of the stir-fry pan rather than using a deep-fat fryer! Do not coat the bread with butter or margarine. Spread thinly instead and the taste will be just as good!

A healthy diet must contain fibre which comes from fruit, vegetables and porridge. There is some evidence that fresh fruit and vegetables taken daily can protect the heart and protect eyesight in old age by providing antioxidants. Some vegetables may have high calories i.e. avocado and some i.e. parsnip may contain sugar however all can be eaten to advantage in moderate amounts (a couple of helpings per week) with no effect on body weight. Fruit and vegetables are important sources of water, vitamins and minerals. If possible, avoid peeling them because the skin contains fibre. Eat raw or cook for the minimum time possible to avoid destroying the vitamins. Where possible use vegetables and fruit that are grown locally to avoid high preservative content. Vegetables and fruit that have been picked at full ripeness offer the biggest health benefits. Garlic contains allicin a substance with anti-viral, anti-fungal, anti-bacterial and antioxidant properties. It has the ability to boost the immune system and prevents the formation of cancer-inducing agents called nitrosamines. It also has anticoagulant properties and both garlic and onions reduces the stickiness of the blood.

- Vitamin A comes from fish and vegetable oils, dairy foods, green vegetables, beetroot and carrots and is important for the immune system, to maintain healthy skin and to prevent night blindness. *It should not be taken as a supplement in pregnancy and should never be taken in excess of the recommended daily amount as liver damage can occur.*

- The B vitamins are necessary for tissue growth, and folic acid and vitamin B_{12} (both are B vitamins) are essential for the proper formation of red blood cells. Most B vitamins are present in yeast, green vegetables, avocado, banana, whole grain foods, fish, meat, poultry and eggs. Beer contains some B vitamins and silicon. B_{12} is present in meat, dairy products and eggs so strict vegetarians need to take B_{12} supplements. High levels of a substance in the body called homocysteine are asssociated with vascular disease including heart disease. Folic acid decreases this. Folic acid also reduces the incidence of spina bifida. Spina bifida occurrence is high in Ireland which is why a folic acid supplement should be taken in the dose prescribed by the GP from the start of pregnancy. The USA has added folic acid to all grain products since 1999. This same procedure may be followed in Ireland in the next few years. Pernicious anaemia is a blood disorder due to B_{12} deficiency which is relatively common in Irish people. B_{12} and folic acid should always be measured together because the true diagnosis of B_{12} deficiency may be missed with serious consequences if folic acid is taken without adequate supplementation with B_{12}. Vitamin B_6 has in some studies been found to reduce the symptoms of pre-menstrual syndrome. **As indicated below for vitamin E, except in special circumstances, it is better to take vitamins as part of the diet rather than as supplements.**

- Vitamin C comes from fresh fruit and supports blood vessels thus helping to prevent bleeding. Sailors in former times did not have fresh fruit on board their boat and often suffered from scurvy which caused bleeding from teeth, skin and other tissues. Recent studies indicate that vitamins C and E may slow the progress of an age-related retinal eye disease called macular degeneration. Avocado contains vitamins C and E and avocados are much cheaper than a take-away!.

- Vitamin D comes from oily fish, eggs, margarine and cheese and is made in the skin from the effect of moderate exposure to the sun. When sun is scarce the diet is the only source. (However this is not a reason to stock up on sun and get sunburnt when the sun is out! The skin must always be protected from excess sun). Vitamin D helps to keep bones healthy. Vitamin D may also reduce the risk of developing diabetes.

- Vitamin E is obtained from spinach, oily fish, nut oil, almonds, sweet peppers, avocado, wholemeal products and egg yolk. Animals lacking this vitamin develop muscular disorders and sterility. Recent research has indicated that vitamin E may help prevent prostate cancer. That research also showed that it was better to take vitamin E from fresh food rather than supplements and this is probably true for all the vitamins. *Vitamin E supplements should not be taken in pregnancy.*

- Vitamin K comes from green vegetables and soya beans and is essential for blood clotting.

Some medical conditions, pregnancy and strict vegetarians do require vitamin supplements.

Vitamins should never be taken in excess as damage to the body may occur.

Glycaemic index (GI) is a measure used for the speed at which carbohydrates are broken down and consequently how fast the blood sugar rises, on a scale of zero to 100. It is important to remember that the glycaemic index of each product is measured separately and since we eat food combinations rather than single items the glycaemic index is only a very rough guide. Also, many different factors affect the GI of the food, including the ripeness of for example the fruit, whether it is solid or juice, and how the food is prepared and combined with other foods. Glycaemic index does not apply to protein or fat because these do not contain carbohydrate.

When eating or preparing meals a good approach to follow is to ensure that no meal raises the blood sugar or fat excessively. To achieve this a few basic principles should be adhered to. For everyday foods choose the so-called 'low glycaemic index' products.[*]

The low glycaemic index foods can of course be combined with moderate amounts of high glycaemic index foods i.e. milk (low GI) with cornflakes (high GI). Table sugar can be added in small amounts to cereal however the addition of fresh fruit will allow reduction of added sugar. Up to 4 teaspoonfuls of added sugar throughout the day are acceptable however if sweet foods such as confectionery (sweets, cakes, pastries) or beer are taken a reduction of added sugar should be made to balance this up. You cannot have your cake and eat sugar too!

Cereal bars are not a substitute for cereal as frequently these contain a lot (33-44%) of sugar (*10% or more is a lot*) and some have a lot (9%) of saturated fat (*5 % of saturated fat is a lot*).

Cakes and sweets are high glycaemic index foods. Again it must be emphasized that cake or biscuit intake should be limited to infrequent occasions, because over a period of time not only will the excess sugar be converted to fat and may increase weight and provoke diabetes, but the fat content is often saturated or hydrogenated (trans) fat both of which should be kept to a minimum, for the health of the heart and brain. Trans fats most often come from margarine-style fats because these are made by solidifying liquid oils with hydrogen. It has been suggested that trans

---

[*]   The low index foods include beans, pasta, porridge, brown or basmati rice, wholegrain bread, low fat milk, boiled potatoes and boiled sweet potatoes. All of these do not significantly raise the blood sugar and tend to decrease LDL- cholesterol (bad cholesterol). Low GI foods must be combined with adequate fibre from fruit and vegetables and in order to slow the passage of food through the stomach they must be combined with some fat. Granary bread, wholegrain and rye bread have lower glycaemic indices than white bread and boiled potato has a lower value compared to baked potato while brown rice is lower than white rice. Eating porridge for breakfast is a wise move since this reduces the appetite and the need for mid-morning snacks.

fats can disrupt the normal messages between brain cells. Butter does not contain trans fats as it is a solid formed by churning milk and no other major additives are added.

Avoid scattering salt liberally on food as most foods, particularly processed foods, already contain salt. Blood pressure elevation may be avoided by restricting salt intake and by increasing potassium intake through eating fruit and vegetables on a regular basis. A moderate amount of alcohol (3 measures or units a day in males and 2 measures in females) can be good for your heart but it is important to remember that excess alcohol from wine, beer or spirits can raise the blood fat levels and trigger high blood pressure, increasing the risk of stroke. Beer contains B vitamins, a useful mineral called silicon and a sugar called maltose. The maltose can cause high fat levels if consumed excessively. Wine like beer should not be consumed in excess of 2-3 units per day.

Have regular meals. Eat food leisurely, do not swallow without savouring the taste. Use small amounts of oil and avoid frying frequently. Drink some water with each meal. Vary the brand of bottled water and use tap water if it is good and pure in your area. Drink coffee and tea in moderation. Both contain antioxidants which are good for health and there is some evidence that coffee can decrease the risk of getting diabetes. Too much coffee or tea however may act as a stimulant because of the caffeine content and may cause tremor or rapid heart beat. Eat plenty of fresh fruit and vegetables. Avoid too many processed foods. Avoid cake or biscuit snacks. Avoid large meals at night. By consuming large meals late at night on a continuous basis reflux of acid may lead to heartburn which is exacerbated by smoking, alcohol, fruit juice and excess weight.

Key sentences: A healthy diet must contain fibre which comes from fresh fruit, vegetables and porridge. When eating or preparing meals a good approach to follow is to ensure that no meal raises the blood sugar or fat excessively.

5

Points To Remember

A bad diet with high saturated fat, high sugar and low fibre content may cause cancer, vascular problems and diabetes. The blood fats (LDL-cholesterol and triglycerides) and blood sugar may rise and increase the stickiness of the blood with the risk of blood clots occurring in the vessels leading to the heart and to the brain. A heart attack or a stroke or both may result. An LDL-cholesterol reduction of about 35% substantially cuts the risk of heart disease. To help your heart it is important also to avoid excessive stress and to stop smoking.

Low density cholesterol or LDL-cholesterol is bad cholesterol.

High density cholesterol or HDL-cholesterol is good cholesterol maintained by a sensible diet and exercise.

Triglycerides are undesirable fats caused by too much carbohydrate particularly added sugars or by too much alcohol.

Free radicals are byproducts in the body, often from poor diet, which can damage your health leading to cancer and allow LDL-cholesterol to accumulate in arteries leading to heart disease. Vitamins A, C, E and the mineral selenium are antioxidants. They can mop up free radicals and thereby help prevent cancer, heart disease and stroke.

Fibre from fruit and vegetables activates the secretion of the bile salts which digest fats and regulate intestinal function. Fibre can block the assimilation of fat thus reducing the risk of atherosclerosis which causes heart, limb and brain disease and fibre lowers the absorption into the bloodstream of carbohydrates, limiting the rise of the blood sugar. Fibre may also limit the effects of toxic food additives. The message is to eat several pieces of fresh fruit and some vegetables every day. Fresh fruit refers to fruit that is not cooked, dried or tinned.

Stewed fruit is also a source of fibre. Fruit can be lightly cooked and small amounts of table sugar or an artificial sweetener such as aspartame can be added.

To lower LDL- cholesterol:

- have lots of fresh fruit and vegetables

- have 1-3 units of alcohol per day if you wish. NEVER DRINK AND DRIVE

- reduce saturated fat and salt

- limit coffee and fizzy drinks

- eat low glycaemic index food*

- have small amounts of olive and vegetable oil

- eat fish once or twice weekly

- have lean meat or poultry and avoid fatty gravy by skimming off the fat.

Some families may have hereditary problems with LDL-cholesterol and may require tablets in association with diet to reduce high levels.

Alcohol should always be taken in moderation and if possible with some food. Moderate alcohol intake (2-3 units daily) increases 'good' HDL-cholesterol and is inversely related with the risk of heart disease but the link with wine alcohol is stronger than with beer alcohol. Red wine contains polyphenols in addition to alcohol. Polyphenols are thought to have antioxidant activity and to reduce the stickiness of blood, both of which have a beneficial action on the heart. Polyphenols are also present in tea, leeks, apples, broccoli, onions, lettuce and cranberries so all of these products are good in moderate amounts. A recent study has found that wine appears to be healthier than beer because wine drinkers tend to eat healthier foods than beer drinkers who often consume excessive processed foods.

---

* The low index foods include beans, pasta, porridge, brown or basmati rice, wholegrain bread, low fat milk, boiled potatoes and boiled sweet potatoes.

Excess or prolonged drinking can cause vitamin B_1 deficiency and can raise the triglycerides and the blood pressure. An intake of more than 2-3 drinks per day may be associated with a higher risk for stroke because of a blood pressure effect. Alcohol consumed without food can on occasions cause a low blood sugar because alcohol inhibits the formation of sugar in the body. A low blood sugar can cause a seizure or fit because brain cells must have sugar for their survival.

Low alcohol drinks contain a lot of calories and should be avoided or taken infrequently.

Asparagus is a natural diuretic (promotes urine secretion). It contains potassium, zinc, selenium and vitamin B.

Avocado which is readily available in all good food stores and cheaper than sweets, fizzy drinks or chips, is a source of 'good' monosaturated oil, vitamins A, C, E and potassium. Added pepper makes it taste delicious. Who would be without one a few times per week?

Bean sprouts contain alfalfa which is a nutritional protein.

Beans of all varieties contain protein, minerals, starch and vitamins. Always cook kidney beans as recommended. Inadequate cooking can lead to toxin accumulation.

The *blueberry* is an excellent source of antioxidants which are good for the body.

Broccoli has antioxidant properties so buy when in season.

Campylobacter are the bacteria that cause a large proportion of food poisoning. To avoid campylobacter contamination it is important to keep food stored properly and avoid contamination of foodstuffs with blood from raw meat or poultry. Defrost food adequately before cooking. Always heat food properly. Water Authorities must always ensure that campylobacter does not contaminate water supplies.

Excessive *coffee* may trigger a syndrome called 'irritable bowel disease'. High caffeine intake from tea and coffee has been linked with high blood pressure in adolescents in certain racial groups. This again emphasizes the need for variation of diet i.e. do not drink tea or coffee throughout the day. Have some water in-between. Coffee is a stimulant so drinking excess may cause restlessness, abnormal heart rhythm and stomach upset. Decaffeinated coffee may not be particularly beneficial since it may cause an increase in bad LDL-cholesterol.

Cooking of food is very important. Boiled and steamed food is far healthier and much more economical than fried food. Fried food not only may contain excessive and denatured fat but during frying harmful particles are found in the air. Ventilation is very important during cooking. Barbecued food if cooked for too long can result in harmful products. Cooking before the coals are ready can cause food to be black on the outside with potential cancer-forming compounds, while inside the food may be raw.

Cranberry juice or products may help to reduce the recurrence of urinary tract infections and may also have preventive effects on gum disease. Sucrose is often added to cranberry products so be moderate with the helping of cranberry sauce or juice!

Crystallised *ginger* helps reduce the nausea of alcohol excess while reminding one that the alcohol should be reduced next time. Crystallised ginger may also be useful for the nausea of 'irritable bowel syndrome', but can contain a lot of sugar and therefore should be taken in small amounts.

Sometimes *drugs* i.e. the contraceptive pill can modify absorption or metabolism of vitamins. This should be mentioned on the drug leaflet. Always read the information that comes with your tablets or injections. If you cannot read, get someone to read this for you.

E 221 is sodium sulphite and is used as a preservative in food. It can cause a dry bitter sensation and can cause allergies. Use local produce where possible to avoid too many preservatives.

E621 is monosodium glutamate which is used as a food additive and can cause headache and nausea.

Eating too little can sometimes be as bad as eating too much. Television can on occasions give the impression that 'no woman can be too thin'. Unfortunately a woman or teenager can become too thin with a disastrously haggard appearance or more serious consequences.

Anorexia nervosa may occur in families, with a history of anorexia in a female parent or a sister of the patient. Anorexia has a high, approximately 15% mortality rate, while 4 out of 10 patients fully recover. Bulimia, often with depression, may be seen in 1% of women in a GP practice. Bulimia often presents in subjects in their twenties or thirties and is most often linked with a traumatic childhood.

Patients with the various eating disorders or suffering with depression, anxiety, obsessive-compulsive disease (OCD) or with seasonal variation of symptoms (Seasonal affective disorder or SAD) all show clinical features of a serotonin dysregulation. Serotonin is a neurotransmitter involved with mood and emotion. Obsessive-compulsive disorder is extreme when compulsive acts cause social or work disruption. In 40% of cases, one or more family members have OCD symptoms however persons with no family history may develop OCD following stress. The use of drugs which modify levels of serotonin are used particularly in bulimia and obsessive disorders. In anorexia, treatment needs to address both physical and psychological problems. Family therapy is often used. Behavioural therapy is perhaps the best treatment at present. Treatment must begin as early as the condition is suspected and family involvement is important.

Although there had been a 20% increase in calls to eating disorder help-lines in Ireland in recent months, the number of eating disorders such as bulimia, compulsive eating and anorexia, all diagnosed mainly in women, may have begun to level off. Like all diseases, prevention is always better than cure. Education about why we need essential substances in our diet can be a useful practice in young children. Parents have an enormous responsibility towards their children and by and large most parents try to assume this and set a good example by sensible eating and appropriate attitude. Self-esteem enhancement for all young adults is important as is a background of normal healthy eating and family pursuits without undue emphasis on diet or body shape. It is important to avoid a series of events leading to eating disorders in the child, which may prove very difficult to treat. If for example a mother has an eating disorder, the child (usually the daughter) may also develop this. If the mother is dissatisfied with her own appearance she must try and deal with this, if necessary with external help, without communicating her opinions to the child. The mother of an anorectic child should be advised not to become or act over-anxious in the child's presence as this behaviour is not conducive to helping the child.

There is some recent research which suggests that eating disorders may be caused by infections which attack the immune system. Antibodies have been found in the blood of subjects with anorexia and bulimia and these conditions may turn out to be autoimmune diseases rather similar to rheumatoid arthritis. Further research will be needed to investigate this possibility which would have enormous implications for treatment.

E. coli 157 may occur in unpasteurized dairy products and uncooked hamburgers. This is a very serious infection. It is important to buy food products particularly meat, from a reputable source.

Food intolerance can be a problem. Lactose is the sugar present in milk. Lactose intolerance is a disorder in which the subject experiences unpleasant stomach or bowel symptoms as a result of taking milk or dairy products. Thorough investigation must be carried out because once a positive diagnosis is made, lactose-free products should be taken. A soya substitute can be used. Calcium and vitamin supplements may also have to be taken. If soya milk is given to babies it must be 'full formula'. Like humans an increasing number of pets have been found to suffer from intolerance to products containing wheat and dairy produce. The offending items may be the human snacks fed to the animals by well-meaning but misguided owners! Refined starch such as is present in white bread and sugar can be eaten occasionally by children and adults but fresh fruit, wholegrain bread, potatoes and brown rice are preferable for a nutritious stable diet and are likely to be more protective for the gut than the refined products.

There is presently no consensus regarding the safety or otherwise of *genetically modified* (GM) products. Foods containing these must be appropriately labelled. GM soya has been available in the US for the past ten years. While there is no evidence from the US that GM foods damage health it is prudent to avoid GM foods during pregnancy until further safety evidence in humans is available.

Ice cream has a relatively low glycaemic index of 35 so although it contains fat (vegetable fat usually) a single scoop twice a week is acceptable. To avoid infection always make sure that the ice-cream is solid and not runny. Sorbet also has a low glycaemic index and low fat so it too can be taken in moderate portions as a dessert.

Lactoferrin is an iron-binding protein which is present in breast milk in quantities 10-20 times greater than in cows' milk. Lactoferrin in association with other proteins strongly inhibits the growth of the E. Coli bacterium so breast feeding may help prevent infection in the newborn baby. Breast feeding is very low in Ireland possibly contributing to our poor overall health relative to other EU countries. Breast feeding must be strongly encouraged.

Listeria can occur in soft cheese and milk. Pregnant women should be warned to avoid soft cheese during pregnancy.

Lycopene is a substance found in tomatoes which may reduce the risk of cancer because of its ant-oxidant properties.

Milk products are an excellent source of calcium and vitamins A and D. Subsidies for school milk should remain and all children encouraged to drink milk and discouraged from regular drinking of fizzy drinks. Neither calcium or vitamins A & D reside in the fat so low fat milk and yoghurt have the same nutrient value as whole milk however whole milk is the preferred product in children.

Nuts are present in marzipan, Worcester sauce, pesto sauce, praline and vegetable oils.

Oily fish such as mackerel contains omega-3 an essential fatty acid which is necessary for the body. Try and avoid frying fish as valuable omega-3 oil may be destroyed. Grilling or oven baking are less destructive. Oily fish can also reduce the stickiness of blood and thus helps to avoid stroke. Fish consumption also reduces the fats called triglycerides which can promote weight gain.

Olive oil helps to reduce LDL, the bad cholesterol.

Peanut allergy is the most serious of the food allergies and those with this condition usually also have asthma and or eczema. Peanut allergy may have arisen in the first year of life through the use of wipes and creams containing peanut oil. Children nowadays are also eating more nuts as part of their diet and while this may be healthy for some children, for others it may not be a good idea. Generally it is advisable to restrict peanuts in the diet until a child is about 6 years old. If there is a definite history of nut allergy, a nut-free diet is advised. Peanut oil is often used in restaurants so eating out involves selection of known nut-free foods. Approximately one quarter of all children with a history of allergy will grow out of this by about 10 years of age.

Phytoestrogens are plant-derived non-steroidal substances found in grains, beans, carrots, spinach, broccoli and soya products. These have weak oestrogen-like activity and may help during the menopause. They also may reduce the risk of certain types of cancer.

Even in the kitchen, *poisons* linger. Polychlorinated biphenyls (PCBs), which in certain circumstances can cause liver and brain damage, linger in the environment for many years because of their low solubility in water even though their use in the manufacture of paints, varnishes and pesticides has been banned. PCBs can be found in very small quantities in dairy products and in fish. If ingested, PCBs can last much longer in some people than others depending on individual metabolism. It is prudent to avoid eating fish caught in local rivers or in inland lakes, however the benefit of eating fish twice a week (once weekly in pregnancy) is far outweighed by any possible risk from PCBs or from mercury in fish. Phthalates which can reduce sperm count or damage the kidney may be found in plastic food wrapping so this should be kept to a minimum. Perfluorinated chemicals which can cause bladder cancer are used in non-stick frying pans so caution is needed not to overheat or overuse the frying pan! It is important to remember however that these toxins are present in very small amounts so while caution is needed continuous worry over frying pans and wrapping is not warranted. Organophosphorus pesticides which also have been used in nerve gas have been banned for many years but are still used in countries needing mosquito control. Traces of these pesticides may contaminate imported meat, fruit and vegetables so make sure that fruit and vegetables are washed before use. One should always be very careful about meat, buying only traceable products and avoiding meat, poultry or fish of uncertain origin. Dioxins from incinerators or burning rubbish can enter the food chain in small amounts in cows' milk and may gradually accumulate in the environment. The way around this is for the appropriate local authority to ensure that advice is sought from the Environmental Protection Agency (EPA) before a licence is granted for commercial incineration and to ensure that incinerators are not built too close to residential properties. People must ensure that rubbish is not burnt in the back garden and that appropriate ventilation is ensured at all times. If you pollute your environment you pollute yourself.

Porridge helps to balance out the blood sugar the morning after drinking alcohol and is always good for the system. It is best however not to drink excessive alcohol!

Red 2G is a synthetic coal tar or azo dye which may cause hyperactivity. Hyperactivity in young children has been linked to food additives such as colorants. Removal of these substances from food and drinks may provide health benefits for children, however there is no conclusive evidence that the additives cause hyperactivity. A lot of foods that contain additives also contain a high sugar content which in itself might have adverse effects. *The prudent action for parents is to buy local produce if possible and to ensure a varied sensible diet for both the children and themselves thus avoiding consumption of excessive additives.*

Salmonella may occur in meat, poultry or eggs. Adequate storing, handling and cooking of these products must take place.

Selenium helps the hair, It is found in eggs and brazil nuts.

Stomach ulcers and stomach cancer in developed countries are now relatively uncommon because the organism responsible for causing ulcers called Helicobacter pylori can be treated effectively by improved hygiene and antibiotics. However it is now known that Helicobacter pylori, a bacterium seen in the human stomach as early as 1875 may actually protect people against disease of the oesophagus or gullet. Cancer of the gullet is rising in most western countries and is often linked to poor lifestyle with smoking and excessive alcohol. It is unknown whether or not the increase in cancer of the gullet is due to poor lifestyle habits or the eradication of the Helicobacter bacterium from the stomach by anti-ulcer treatment. The idea that microbes can be eaten to aid human health has focused on bacteria that make yoghurt and cheese. These are called probiotics or friendly bacteria. Probiotics that contain a plant sugar that feeds the good gut bacteria may aid digestion, and may be useful when a course of antibiotics or anti-ulcer treatment has taken out the friendly bacteria as well as any bad bacteria. Probiotics may also boost immunity. Although there are many yoghurts and fruits drinks on the market which are said to contain probiotics it is likely that there are not enough good bacteria present in these since a lot of the bacteria are broken down in the stomach before reaching the gut. Some studies indicate that a capsule preparation of probiotics may prevent their destruction in the stomach and allow some of the probiotic to reach the gut.

Sugar is found as fructose (the natural sugar in fruit) or is present as added sugar such as glucose /glucose syrup (jams/sweets), maltose (sugar in beer) and sucrose (or table sugar). One plain biscuit contains half a teaspoon of sugar, a fruit yoghurt can contain several teaspoonfuls and a portion of sugar-coated cereals contains about 3 teaspoonfuls. Processed food therefore may contain a lot of added sugar. In order not to exceed the recommended 50-70 gram per day which includes sugar already present in food plus any added sugar, avoid using the sugar bowl excessively. Added sugar should not exceed around 1 oz or 4 teaspoonfuls per day. Try and get all the sugar you need from fresh fruit!

Vinegar can be used to: clean the house, give whites a freshly laundered look, get rid of weeds and in cooking. It can help avoid overuse of synthetic cleansers.

A well-balanced diet should contain adequate *vitamins and minerals*. Proper food preparation should ensure that vitamins are not destroyed i.e. vitamin A can be destroyed by excessive frying. Even healthy vegetable oils can become poisonous if heated to a high temperature. Vegetable oils have high levels of linoleic acid which is good for you however if the oil is heated excessively or for too long, or is re-heated, toxic compounds called noneals are formed. These toxins have been implicated in heart disease, stroke, Parkinson's disease, Alzheimer's disease and liver disease. The message is to avoid frying excessively and re-heating oils. Chips should not be eaten frequently.

There should be no need for the healthy individual to take vitamin supplements. However in some circumstances i.e. in strict vegetarians or in medical conditions where food is not absorbed properly, both vitamins and mineral supplements are required. In a strict vegetarian diet, vitamin B_{12} and some iron supplements will need to be taken since red meat usually provides these although some B_{12} is present in dairy products. Iron from meat is called haem iron. Iron from bread, beans, fruit vegetables and eggs is called non-haem iron. Eggs, nuts, leafy vegetables, peas and beans are all good sources of iron but vegetables need to be taken with foods rich in vitamin C (fresh fruit, potatoes) in order to ensure adequate iron absorption. Sweet and sour combinations of fruit and vegetables taste good and can increase iron absorption.

80% of *vitamin* D comes from the sun effect on skin. 15 minutes daily of moderate sun exposure is adequate and avoid mid-day sun. Vitamin D levels decrease in all of us during the winter months when sunlight is scarce so vitamin D must be obtained from the diet. Recent studies have indicated that we all probably need to replenish vitamin D stores during the winter months. Eating salmon, herring or mackerel, eggs and bread will replenish stores. People of Asian origin who come to live in the UK or Ireland may become vitamin D deficient because of absence of sunlight and inadequate vitamin D intake in the diet. Inadequate vitamin D can lead to bone problems called rickets in children or osteomalacia in adults. Asian people, the elderly, pregnant or breastfeeding women may need to take vitamin D supplements if their diet is unsatisfactory. Subjects suffering with absorption problems or taking certain medication may also need to take supplements. Smoking affects the metabolism of drugs and vitamins and may cause decreased levels of vitamin D.

Everyone should try and drink a couple of glasses of *water* (still or sparkling) per day. Water is a very important item in our diet and we are lucky to have access to good pure water. Long may this be the case so remember to use water wisely. Never waste it, since if third world countries had access to sufficient clean water a huge amount of their illnesses would be non-existent.

Sugar-free *yoghurt* fermented with streptococcal and lactobacillus bacteria has been found to reduce the effects of bad breath. Sulphide compounds create bad breath. Plain yoghurt tastes great with and without fruit and may also be useful for fresh breath.

Key sentences: The prudent action for parents is to ensure a varied sensible diet for both the children and themselves, thus avoiding consumption of excessive additives. Self-esteem enhancement for all young adults is important as is a background of normal healthy eating and family pursuits without undue emphasis on diet or body shape.

6

Exercise

Physical activity is linked with longevity. You do not need to go to the gym to exercise. You certainly can go and 'pump iron' but other forms of exercise can prove equally satisfactory and moderate aerobic exercise such as walking is just as effective as intense exercise. Exercise needs to be regular and sustained rather than vigorous. Work-outs at home can lead to injuries because of over-ambitious routines so a gradual build-up is advisable. In many people, lack of exercise rather than eating too much is responsible for excess weight. Choose the activity that suits you. The gardaí have now got bike units which have been successful in tackling some anti-social behaviour. The unit seems to work well in conjunction with other units and the biking should also be beneficial in keeping the officers fit.

Exercise has a beneficial effect not only on the overall weight but also affects the distribution of weight, with less weight gain but also less accumulation of weight on the abdomen ('belly'). Subjects with big stomachs due to fat accumulation have a greater risk of heart disease and diabetes than thin individuals or subjects with fat accumulation on the buttocks. If you are trying to lose weight, increasing your exercise and changing to a sensible diet will be more effective than diet alone. Genes are the 'units of heredity' which are involved in passing on biological information from one generation to the next. Despite the influence of our genes the environment is always important. Even though your parents are fat that does not mean that you must be fat. You can defy your genes by exercise and sensible eating! Hundreds of genes in the thighs are activated in regular cycle training, making the body more switched on to exercise. Exercise is associated with a lower risk of death from coronary artery disease, a lower blood pressure and probably improves quality of life. Exercise may also have a role in stress reduction and may boost the immune system. Even moderate exercise may reduce the impact of stress on the immune system.

Skeletal muscle can adopt quite quickly to different levels of activity. Muscular activity ensures that the body mobilizes adaptive mechanisms to meet the heart and lung requirements. Even the prospect of exercise can start this process. You will notice during brisk walking that you become warm and breathe faster. This is normal. However an individual unaccustomed to habitual physical activity has a 50-100% increase in the risk of heart attack or death when undertaking vigorous exercise. Heavy exertion should therefore be avoided especially for those who are unfit. Exercise must be commenced gradually with a small daily increase, as breathing and muscles must get used to the extra work. In the UK, several deaths occurred during the 2005 Great North Run. At least 2 of these people were less than 35 years of age and all were less than 60 years. Most of these people had experience of running in marathons. The big factor was the heat of the day. Although water was supplied, dehydration which can go unnoticed at least initially may well have played a major part in the deaths. It is important to ensure adequate but not excessive hydration at all times. If exercising vigorously, particularly in hot weather, it is wise to drink a couple of glasses of water. If planning to run in a marathon speak to your GP for advice before you do so.

The rule must be, where feasible, to walk everywhere. Comfortable shoes are essential for optimal exercise. By persistently wearing narrow shoes you may end up with a bunion which is a swelling over the junction between the big toe and the metatarsal or foot bone, with resulting deformity. Climb stairs rather than take the escalator and avoid sitting in front of the television for prolonged periods. Walking, gardening, vacuuming, window cleaning and mowing the lawn are all excellent practical ways of exercising, using up between 3 and 7 kilocalories per minute so gradual decreases in blood fat and blood sugar levels can be expected. Bicycling, swimming and dancing are also excellent forms of exercise but injury from bicycle falls must be guarded against by care on the roads and wearing appropriate gear including a luminous or other suitable identification at night. Intense cycling is great exercise but prolonged periods of cycling on bikes with long narrow saddles can lead to decreased blood flow and numbness in a man's penis. More comfortable saddles should cure this problem. If you go swimming always make sure that there is someone with you, never swim in unsafe waters and ensure that help can be summoned quickly should this be needed either for yourself or for other swimmers. As an island nation most Irish people should be able to swim so if you cannot swim take up lessons if available in your area. Avoid swimming in lakes. Diving centres are only for those expert in the sport and these probably should be regulated. Avoid alcohol intake if you plan to swim, surf or drive a cruiser. Obviously it is unwise to go hill-walking in thunder and lightening conditions or if you have taken alcohol so common sense must prevail.

Any form of exercise which is not dangerous must be encouraged. Soccer is a great sport but there are a lot of injuries reported from this. Fortunately they are not usually serious. Many young men who have played hurling have been left with no teeth and many young men who have played rugby have suffered loss of power and movement due to damage to the nerves. Accidents in rugby often result from dangerous tackles rather than the scrum. Sport must not be a destructive exercise and savage tackles must be heavily penalized.

Tennis, squash, racquet ball are all very acceptable forms of exercise however eye protection should be worn particularly in squash and racquet ball. The use of helmets in hurling is now advised in order to reduce eye injury. Water-skiing can cause injury to the ears or to the back so it is important not to mistake the need for exercise with excessive risk taking, particularly if one has not got experience in a particular sport.

Research has shown that there is a negative correlation between a measure of physical fitness called oxygen uptake and a measure of size called waist-hip ratio. The waist-hip ratio gives similar information to the waist measurement described previously. The more fit you are, the lower the waist-hip ratio. The bigger the waist-hip ratio the greater the accumulation of abdominal fat or apple-shape which is bad for the health and particularly bad for the heart. Regular exercise can reduce abdominal fat accumulation. Exercise has a beneficial effect not only on the blood fats but on the blood sugar. Many studies have shown that regular participation in aerobic physical activities as described above, is part of a healthy lifestyle which contributes to the prevention of heart disease and diabetes mellitus.

Exercise not only stimulates bone formation thus helping to avoid osteoporosis later on in life but by careful exposure of the skin to sunlight, vitamin D supplies are replenished. Exercise stimulates endorphins which are physiological opioids. Endorphins can give a feeling of well-being, however there is no need to exercise too strenuously in order to achieve a 'high'! Sport is said to encourage self-discipline and team spirit however aggression must be avoided. Participation in exercise at school should be strongly encouraged but never forced upon a child. Encourage children to walk to school if this is feasible or to use public transport. There is nothing more conducive to obesity in children and adults than parents taking children to school by car. In a recent UK survey, 67% of parents did not notice that their children were getting fatter! Walking everywhere possible must be encouraged for everyone and the use of the car limited to necessary journeys. Advise children not to accept lifts in anyone else's car either! Children should not be encouraged to use children's equipment in gyms. Active exercise while playing in safe non-vandalized drug-free surroundings should be encouraged. Always know where and with whom your child is playing.

The Adkins diet significantly decreases carbohydrate intake. This may reduce energy stores in the heart leading to problems when exercising. It is important not to exclude any substance from the diet but always to follow a sensible pattern of eating. Never take any form of recreational drug or performance-enhancing drug prior to exercise. Heart arrhythmias or sudden death may result.

During exercise the fluid drunk should be to replace water only, unless the person has been taking part in endurance activities lasting up to two hours or more when sodium, chloride and possibly some magnesium might need replenishment. The perceived need for extra energy may cause some individuals to drink a high sugar content liquid. This would be counterproductive and may result in drawing water from the body back into the stomach in order to dilute the drink sufficiently for absorption, thus causing the body to dehydrate even more.

While going to the gym for exercise is the choice for many people, excessive workout in the gym is both unnecessary and dangerous. Damage to the brain and the heart can occur with over-enthusiastic workouts. After a certain age, osteoarthritis of the joints of the neck may occur or the blood vessels may become less elastic. Vigorous neck movements can cause impaired circulation to the brain tissue particularly in the older subject. Dizziness, brief unconsciousness, temporary or on occasions permanent loss of function in parts of the anatomy i.e. hand or side of the body with a resulting stroke, may occur. Choose walking as your exercise if you can walk well. If your walking ability is limited choose non-vigorous stretching exercise and discuss this with your GP. At any age it is wise not to jump out of bed in the morning but to proceed at a gradual pace. This is particularly important in people with blood pressure problems. As we age the joints tend to get stiff. Small exercises can be practised in bed i.e. opening and shutting the hands and similarly with the feet. When exercising by performing hip and pelvic exercises it is important to be careful of one's back by building up the exercises gradually. Stretching exercise may be useful for people with stiff lower backs and with limited flexibility of the muscles controlling the buttocks. While pre-exercise stretching is not always necessary, never rush into a new exercise without appropriate lead-in and training if necessary!

Elasticated knee supports (available in general stores or pharmacies) are excellent for knee strain or arthritis of the knee but obviously may not be fully remedial if the knee has more extensive damage, when medical advice may be necessary. Tennis elbow causes pain on the outside (thumb side) of the lower arm (forearm) starting below the elbow and getting worse on grip tightening. This can occur from a variety of repetitive activities in the home or in the garden. It occurs most often in the middle-aged individual whose tendon instead of stretching, tears. In the acute painful stage some ice may be soothing. The lesion may take three to four months to heal. During this time normal activity should probably be encouraged. An exercise to stretch the injured tendon may help healing although it may not speed up the natural recovery time. This exercise consists of holding the arm straight out in front with the fingers

57

pointing downwards towards the ground. Rotate the palm inwards with the thumb pointing away from you. This can be repeated several times daily.

Exercise is important in all individuals and can be performed according to each individual's ability. In some individuals asthma can be induced or made worse by exercise because of water loss and nervous mechanisms which can cause constriction of the airways. Adequate pre- exercise medication should control the exercise-induced airway constriction. Subjects with asthma can participate in sport at the highest level provided the asthma is managed properly with a suitable combination of inhalers.

Diabetic patients can if fit to do so, participate in any form of exercise. It is wise to discuss any new activity with your GP and to begin gradually. The benefit from exercise is two-fold. The heart and circulatory system in general benefit and the blood sugar benefits as shown by a decrease in value immediately and in the long-term. If you are using insulin, an appropriate snack with or without insulin reduction may be necessary to avoid too big a drop in blood sugar following exercise.

Remember that just thirty minutes of exercise every day, whether this is continuous or intermittent, reduces the risk of heart disease and may prevent the onset of diabetes. The activity level of muscle has been found to influence several genes that keep us healthy indicating that under-activity has a negative effect on the body. In order to achieve good health, exercise must contribute a major amount to our lifestyle.

There have been two recent reports of goal posts falling on and killing young football players. This type of horrific event must remind us all that any equipment used during exercise or sporting events must be in good order and must be inspected on a regular basis. Goal posts in sports grounds should be inspected to ensure stability and freedom from defect. Children should be warned not to tamper with any equipment.

Be vigilant of your feet. Do not cut toe-nails too short and always examine the soles of your feet after exercise. Whether you walk, hike or exercise in the gym do not wear the same trainers every day. Use a spare pair of shoes to give the original shoes time to breathe and get rid of built-up debris which may lead to infection. Dirty gym towels may spread methicillin-resistant staphylococcus aureus (MRSA) so always bring your own clean towel with you and avoid preventable infection.

Key sentence: Thirty minutes of exercise every day, whether this is continuous or intermittent, reduces the risk of heart disease and may prevent the onset of diabetes.

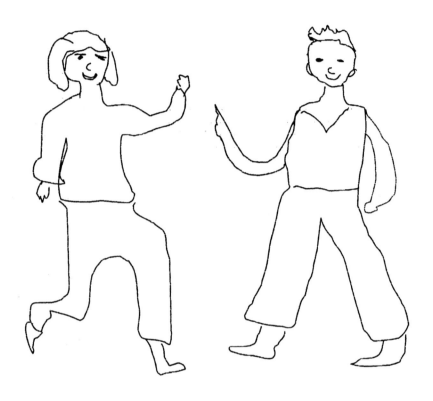

WE KEEP FIT BY DANCING

7

In The Home

Most accidents occur in the home. Accidents at home place a heavy burden on A & E departments, yet most of these are potentially preventable. A recent survey has indicated that 40% of X-rays are unnecessary so keeping healthy and preventing accidents should help us all to avoid unnecessary radiation. In Ireland there are approximately 1500 unintentional accidents per year. A considerable proportion of acute hospital beds are used in the treatment of unintentional injuries including falls, inhalation of toxic substances, poisoning, suffocating, drowning, burns, electrocution, a strain or a cut or being struck by an object. Falls account for 47% of injury admissions to Irish hospitals. Recent research has found that August particularly on a Saturday in early afternoon is the most likely time for accidents to occur in Irish homes. Fewer accidents occurred in the winter months which is somewhat surprising since in other countries Christmas appears to be the peak season for accidents in the home. Accidental injury is a particularly important cause of disability and death in childhood. Items associated with accidents include sports equipment, tools and kitchen utensils, hot food, toys, floors and footwear.

There are three factors involved in accident occurrence:

- The person,

- the causative agent

- the environment.

A smoke alarm must be installed in the home. This is cheap, simple to install and life saving. Fires caused by cigarettes are the biggest cause of house fire deaths. A total of 39 people died in domestic fires in Ireland in 2004, an increase of two on the figure for 2003. According to the National Safety Council no smoke alarm was fitted to four out of five fatal house fires in Ireland during 2004. Many people have lost their lives because of the absence of a smoke detector. Make it as important in your home as the TV because it really is much more important! Test the alarm periodically to ensure that the battery is functioning. A small fire blanket which can be purchased in a hardware store is very useful for users of chip pans. While frequent use of chip pans with all the fat therein is never advisable, if the fat should take fire the blanket can be thrown over the pan to quench the fire. A wet cloth can also be used. **Do not die because a smoke alarm was not purchased, The smoke alarm is cheaper than cigarettes or a take-away. Never smoke in bed!**

The younger the child the greater the parental responsibility. It is important to foresee and avoid objects or situations that can cause injury. Children are inquisitive. Prepare to be one step ahead of them. Close rooms where items of furniture are heavy and could be unstable. Recently a child was killed when he opened the drawers of a large cupboard which subsequently fell on top of him. Children should be trained to keep clear of the cooker. Pot handles should be turned inwards, away from moving objects. Electricity should be up to date and fault-free. If in any doubt call an experienced electrician. The money will be well-spent. The child should be trained to respect the electricity and never to insert objects into sockets. Tablets, detergents or other liquids must be kept in areas where children cannot get them. Death from accidental poisoning is a real tragedy.

Sensible shoes should be worn to avoid falling down the stairs or tripping. Always tie shoelaces properly. Tiles should be non-slip with a good steady surface. Mats should not be placed in positions where a person can trip or fall. Oven gloves or a suitable alternative must be used to lift hot objects. Never take a chance and think that you do not need them. When cutting vegetables and meat, be careful to use a cutting board or suitable surface and use cutting strokes away from the body. Knives must be treated with care. Never leave a sharp knife in a position where it can cause body damage. Be careful of cocktail sticks. Small sharp bits of these may be swallowed with fatal consequences.

Electric kettles, microwave ovens and computers may all have small electromagnetic fields. Some people may be more sensitive than others to electricity. It is important to unplug these devices when not in use and not to use them continuously. Mobile phones should also be used with care especially by children. Do not talk on any phone for long periods, oblivious to the fact that your child has just found your iron tablets and has swallowed them.

Gas is a wonderful clean source of energy inside and outside the home. All fossil (gas, oil and coal) sources of energy can cause carbon monoxide poisoning if there is inadequate ventilation. Always ensure that the central heating boiler is serviced properly and that the flue is not blocked. Year after year, around the world, deaths from carbon monoxide poisoning continue to occur. Sometimes the fault lies with the householder who in cold weather closes the air vents so that in a double glazed room there may be little or no ventilation with a possible build-up of carbon monoxide. The acute symptoms of carbon monoxide poisoning are subtle and include headache, problems with vision, sickness and diarrhoea, stomach pains and general lack of energy. The subject affected may not realise that the home ventilation is to blame and may seek a doctor's opinion. Often the diagnosis is completely missed and an erroneous diagnosis of viral infection made. Carbon monoxide poisoning can cause neurological signs with coma and convulsions and death may occur during sleep. Chronic carbon monoxide poisoning can lead to Parkinson's disease with all its attendant morbidity. With all fossil fuels it is vital to take precautions and not to risk death through negligence. Together with appropriate servicing of equipment and good ventilation, a carbon monoxide alarm is a simple and inexpensive additional measure which is available from reputable hardware stores.

Formaldehyde solution is no longer used as a disinfectant however, in gaseous form, it may be present as a preservative in resins, newsprint and in chipboard. It is always important to have good house ventilation.

Vents must not be closed and the house should be aired regularly. Spider plants can also be useful to absorb any residues.

If gas cylinders are used in the home, follow instructions for storage and use carefully.

Electric shock can occur in the home. Do not touch the victim if he is in contact with the electric current. Always try to switch off the mains or pull out the plug. Push the victim away from the electric source using a non-metallic object i.e. something wooden like a brush or chair.

Always ensure that tablets are kept away from children. The ease with which 'controlled' drugs can be bought online has been highlighted in the UK where many young people have committed suicide by easy access to a variety of drugs. What is not known as yet is the extent of such abuse. The International Narcotics Control Board has warned that global sales of illegal and prescription-only drugs are rising on the internet. There are an estimated 2000 sites selling drugs directly to the consumer. Teenagers with credit card access can go online and get tablets through the post after filling in a questionnaire, often with false information. While the problem may not be a major one at present it is important that education at home and, at school should stress that any tablet can kill if not adequately supervised. It is important that internet service providers remove illegal sites from their servers and that parents keep an eye on the computer and ensure that access to the internet is used appropriately.

No drug is 100% safe for everybody. Any drug is capable in certain individuals of causing any type of reaction. At present adverse reaction cannot usually be predicted. In the future it is likely that it will be possible to prescribe drugs tailor-made so to speak, for each individual, but at present our pharmacogenetic knowledge is not adequate for this. It may however soon be possible using a blood test, to say if a tablet is suitable for a particular person. Ensure that only the person for which the tablets have been prescribed has access to the tablets. Remember that paracetamol is a very useful drug but taking even one more than the stated safe dose can be lethal and may cause liver failure and death. *Alcohol can interact with paracetamol so the two should not be combined.* Aspirin is also a very useful drug but can on occasions, in certain people, produce almost any theoretical reaction. Bleeding is a well recognised complication in some individuals while asthmatic attacks can be precipitated in patients with and without a history of asthma.

Eczema in various forms can be caused by a variety of home irritants including stress. Irritation of the skin can occur in any individual depending on the duration of exposure, concentration of the irritant and the hydration of the skin. Avoid any known causative factors and use cotton next to the skin as it is non-irritating. Topical primrose oil products can reduce dryness and itching. Anti-histamine or anti-inflammatory tablets may be necessary to reduce swelling.

Irritation is different to an allergic reaction. An allergic reaction is an immune reaction directed against a specific allergen often in very small amounts. In recent years there has been a rise in allergy incidence possibly because of the existence of super-clean homes in which young children's immune system cannot develop properly. In a person with a history of allergy to a substance, further contact almost invariably produces a rash or more serious reaction. Severe allergic reactions are not common but can be life-threatening. More than 90% of severe allergic reactions are caused by nuts, fish, wheat, milk, eggs and soya. Peanut allergy may be quite common and involves nut elimination from the diet. Severe allergic reactions can also occur to insect bites or latex rubber. It is important to find out exactly what is causing the allergy in order to avoid unnecessary elimination of items from the diet. Children with allergy can have a poor quality of life following uncertainty with food content so it essential to ensure food label content is adequate and complete. Children brought up with pets from an early age have been found to be less likely to suffer from allergies. The overuse of cleansing agents is not advisable.

While over-hygienic measures should be avoided and indeed children may develop a more efficient immune system by exposure to dirt, teddy bears should if possible be washed from time to time to avoid unsavoury smells and infection.

Recycle old newspapers. Avoid commercial cleaning fluid. Use a damp cloth for dusting and clean floors with hot water. Do not be over-zealous. If necessary, disinfectants and cleansers should be used in small amounts. Vinegar is as good as purpose-bought cleaners. Lemon juice is good for removing red wine, blood, grass stains and limescale.

Soda water is good for coffee stains. Aerosols may cause headache and depression since they emit volatile organic compounds so do not drench the house with aerosols to cover up cooking or smoking smells. Open the windows for a short period instead and most important of all – stop smoking!

Subjects who are prone to anaphylactic attacks should carry adrenaline for immediate injection should this be necessary in a severe allergic reaction. The Irish Anaphylaxis Campaign was set up some time ago to try and ensure that nobody dies from allergies.

A First Aid kit is useful. While it is hoped that it will not be needed it is important to be able to deal with minor cuts and ailments. If a deep cut is sustained it must be kept clean and bleeding minimised by appropriate pressure. Pressure cannot be sustained with safety for an indefinite period so it is important to seek medical help if bleeding continues. The cut may require stitches and a tetanus shot if this has not been given in the previous ten years. Even minor eye injuries can lead to infection. Do not touch the eye or any contact lens. A sterile pad (or clean pad if sterile dressing not available) is gently placed over the injured eye. The eye must then be examined by the Eye A & E.

Head injuries, especially if accompanied by unconsciousness, must have medical attention.

If a member of the house has a cold avoid close contact until this subsides. Avoid smoking and causing discomfort to other household members who do not smoke. Remember children must not be exposed to cigarettes or cigarette smoke. It may affect their health for the rest of their lives.

Any of us could be faced with an emergency in the home. A short but concise course in first aid and medical emergencies is a very instructive and useful way of aiding members of your household. It is important to obtain the correct information from a reputable source for immediate action in an emergency. A list of such courses should be available from your local information centre or library. Prevention of accidents however is always the best approach.

Key sentence: Most accidents occur in the home

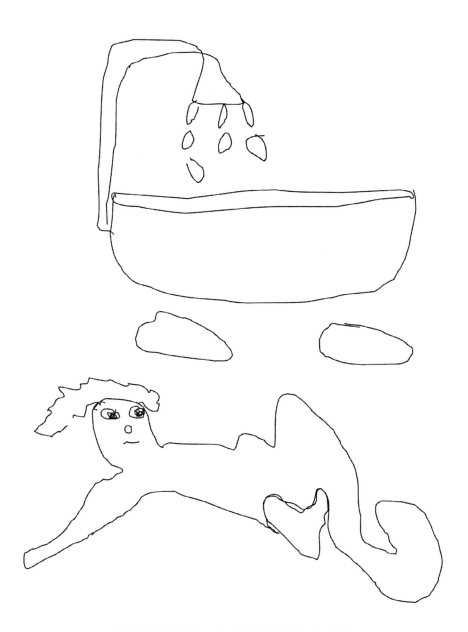

BEWARE OF SLIPPERY FLOORS

8

In The Environment

Traffic congestion, rubbish and illegal dumps are poisoning our once clean environment and polluting our rivers, our fish and our wonderful wildlife. Climate change will cause high ground levels of ozone which will affect our health and plant health. Massive industrial sludge spillages are occurring too frequently, with incalculable damage to marine life. Chemicals released into the sea may be altering the sex of fish, with ovarian tissue being found in the testes of the male fish. If we pollute the fish we pollute ourselves.

Our environment has been exploited by reckless dumping and lack of foresight. The waste is increasing yearly by 10% so some quick entrepreneurial ideas are necessary to avoid the full island becoming a cauldron of dumping and waste. Why are we fouling the country and why do we have a 'throw-away ' mentality? Unfortunately it is due to gaps in wider education and little imagination or ability to reuse items. While there is a 'throw-away' mentality a large proportion of people are reluctant to pay service charges to deal with the waste. 60% of those fined for littering have not paid their fines. There is some good news however regarding recycling and reuse. The old Zetor tractors that had been used in Ireland for more than 50 years are now being sold to farmers in eastern Europe who know how to repair them. Shops are now obliged to take old electronic equipment. More people, 51% versus 40% in 2000, are recycling at least some of their domestic waste. Recycling services should now become more widely available.

Fish is a great and very important food source, however the oceans may soon yield few fish if measures to clean up our seas and oceans and to avoid over-fishing, are not put in place in Ireland and other fishing countries. A long-term vision is needed. There has been a lot of publicity regarding sea pollution which may cause organic mercury to be present in small amounts, in fish. Organic mercury is more toxic than the gaseous inorganic mercury present in old blood pressure measuring equipment. The usefulness and safety of an item must always be looked at from a benefit risk point of view. The benefit versus risk of eating fish has been looked at both by the European Union (EU) and the World Health Organization (WHO). The conclusion is that consumption of fish once or twice a week is beneficial and has a positive benefit risk ratio. In pregnancy it is recommended that fish is eaten once weekly. It is also important to be aware that Ireland eats less fish per capita than our healthier Nordic neighbour Sweden who because of paper and logging industries would have higher organic mercury in the surrounding seas and inland lakes, compared to Ireland.

New EU laws which oblige companies to test chemicals for their ability to cause cancer or asthma should soon be in place. Appropriate regulation for all pharmaceutical and industrial effluents must also be enforced, to ensure that water supplies are kept free from contamination and that organic mercury toxicity or disruptive hormonal effects do not affect the food chain.

Every year many needless deaths are lost at sea and in the fishing and agriculture sectors. Farmers, fisherman and seafarers need to pay great attention to health and safety and to take advice where necessary. The Irish Water Safety has emphasized the need to service and check personal and communal flotation devices, such as lifejackets, regularly. Wear and tear at the folds, straps and fastenings should be examined. Gas bottles on inflatable lifejackets should be full, fitted correctly and have no signs of corrosion. Lifejackets should never be used as cushions. Fishermen should ensure the sea-worthiness of their boats and all must know how to swim. The Department of Communications, Marine and Natural Resources and the Irish Coast Guard have produced a booklet regarding lifejacket maintenance and these are available free of charge. The hazards of tractors have been mentioned many times in the media and in Health and Safety reports. Anyone using a tractor must ensure that adequate training has been obtained to drive carefully, that all safety precautions are observed and that the rules of the road are adhered to.

Accidental deaths on farms have remained high for several years. There were 17 deaths on farms in 2005 and 2 of these were children, compared to 13 in 2004. The farmer has to try and anticipate where danger lies in an effort to prevent a further increase in these numbers. That is not always easy since he must prevent hazard to himself, his family, his workers and his animals. It is important to remember that for the farmer, the slurry pit could be a potential heart hazard. The slurry pit gives off sulphur dioxide which can be damaging to the heart. As with all noxious fumes adequate ventilation is necessary. Leaflets are available regarding the slurry pit and its potential dangers, from local Health and Safety Executive personnel. Depression may be more common amongst the farming community than amongst other workers. Farming has changed considerably, with intense farming methods and large co-operatives replacing traditional farming methods. This has inevitably a negative impact on many small landowners and it is debatable whether it has benefited the consumer. Farmers may need to consider producing crops for bio-fuels in order to survive. This may introduce a new aspect to life in rural areas and could be a stimulus to a more varied lifestyle. Ireland has a very low percentage of its farmland converted to organic farming. Organic farming with benefit to the animals, the environment, the farmers and to the consumers should perhaps be pursued more intensely.

In the environment there are small amounts of synthetic chemicals to which we are exposed, yet relatively little is known about their risk to health. It is important to be aware of the hazards and possibility of absorption through the skin and by inhalation, of chemicals including pesticides. Care needs to be taken when crop spraying of plants with pesticides, in order to ensure that no health risk is sustained by the sprayer or by people in the surrounding areas. In some countries apples are sprayed up to 18 times per year with multiple chemicals. An apparently perfect apple may not be as healthy as a windfall from unsprayed orchard trees. Other fruits such as strawberries and vegetables such as carrots, parsnips and celery require less spraying. It is important to wash all fruit and vegetables before consuming them. Gloves, mask and protective head and body gear should be worn at all times in noxious or hazardous situations. Beware of pesticides left in the garden shed. Make sure that children or depressed individuals do not have access to these. If you do use a pesticide make sure that you take advice regarding the effect of this on the environment as in some cases residues remain in the soil for many years. People who use pesticides are at a significantly higher risk of developing Parkinson's disease. Inhaled material causes the most damage. Use gloves to handle pesticides, wear a mask over the nose and mouth and always wash your hands after use.

Dioxins from incinerators or burning rubbish can enter the food chain in small amounts in cows' milk and may gradually accumulate in the environment. Dioxins can cause cancer. People must realise that by burning rubbish they expose themselves, their families and neighbours to cancer-causing substances. Appropriate local authorities must take advice from the Environmental Protection Agency (EPA) before granting a licence for commercial incineration and must not allow incinerators to be built within a certain distance of residential properties. Rules to ensure that people do not burn rubbish in their backyard must be strictly enforced.

Air quality can affect people suffering with airway or lung disease. The burning of coal in large amounts releases sulphur dioxide. Petrol and diesel engines give off carbon monoxide, oxides of nitrogen and organic compounds. Unventilated farm silos where green crops undergo fermentation for use as animal fodder can give off nitrogen oxides which can cause acute or chronic lung disease. Sunlight can form ozone from the nitrogen oxides. Ozone and nitrogen oxides can be found in the environment during electric or gas welding. Ozone may be formed in and around electrical equipment, in air and water-purifying devices, around printing inks and copying devices which use powerful ultraviolet (UV) light sources. Ozone can cause chest pain, persistent cough, sore throat and nosebleeds and dryness of the eyes and throat. Ensure good ventilation. The permitted levels of all these pollutants are regulated by the EU. Overall the air quality in Ireland is satisfactory however the build-up of traffic in our cities is a cause for concern and will need to be altered by removing cars from city centres and using alternatives to petrol and diesel.

Phthalates may leach out of plastics, fabrics and rainwear. They are also present in some creams, soaps, perfumes, tobacco smoke and car exhausts. Phthalates affect sexual differentiation in unborn male animals and may decrease sperm quality in young male animals. Exposure of the unborn male to organochlorine pesticides which are now banned, has been linked to lower fertility and testicular cancer in the mature animal. PCBs (polychlorinated biphenyls) and mercury will be present in the environment for many years. If eaten by animals these chemicals tend to lodge in fat depots. By avoiding the recycling of contaminated fats through the food fed to farmed salmon and to pigs and chickens, much could be done to decrease both PCBs and mercury in the environment. There is a need for a more comprehensive surveillance of health effects due to environmental chemicals. A list of these chemicals should be available to farmers and if necessary to the general public.

There has been some controversy over whether fluoride should continue to be added to water supplies. Although fluoride may strengthen teeth, other bone problems such as fluorosis may arise. The US EPA has questioned its safety on the grounds that the metabolism of fluoride in water has not been fully evaluated. Most European countries ceased fluoridation in the 1970s. Many dentists in Ireland are not in favour of fluoridation. A recent forum in Ireland to review this practice concluded that at the maximum permitted level of fluoride in drinking water of one part per million, human health is not adversely affected and that the practice should continue as a public health measure. This decision will be reviewed in the near future.

Radon is produced by the radioactive decay of radium which exists in varying amounts in all soil and rocky areas. Radon gas can cause cancer of the lung even in non-smokers, however the risk of developing lung cancer in high radon environments is increased in smokers. The Radiological Protection Institute of Ireland (RPII) has stated that radon gas is responsible for up to 200 deaths a year from lung cancer, with the majority of these deaths occurring in smokers. Those who are living in a high radon area should arrange for a sample of house air to be sent for analysis to the Radiological Institute. If this shows that substantial radon is present, advice on ventilation improvement can be obtained. New homes now have a requirement to be made gas-proof by an upgraded damp-proof membrane.

Asbestos may still be present in the home, in old buildings and on construction sites. Asbestos has been used in the manufacture of fire blankets, ironing boards, brake pads, and asbestos lagging has been used for insulating pipes, in ceiling tiles and in older central heating systems. The danger to health arises from exposure to asbestos fibres. It is essential to ensure that you are protected, in any environment likely to have asbestos fibres. If working on a building site or demolition area always ensure that you ask the site manager regarding this. It is his duty to be aware of the presence or not, of asbestos. If you think that in the past you worked near to or with asbestos-related products, it is important to explore that possibility for health and monetary reasons. There are definite criteria based on a combination of medical history, examination and tests including chest X-ray and other imaging, which can establish if you have been exposed to asbestos in previous employment.

Irish people consistently fail to heed the risk of sunburn, and subject themselves needlessly to the high risk of skin cancer. Ensure that sunscreen and where appropriate, head cover are used by all when the sun is out. If you are allergic to sunscreen a waterproof version without para-aminobenzoic acid (PABA) is available. There is nothing more sad than to see a person with a bald head or a young fair-skinned child walk along under the painful glare of the sun with no head or skin protection.

While cutting trees, be aware of small branches that may damage the eye. Always have a pair of goggles (glasses offer some protection but the glass could get damaged with ensuing injury to the eyeball) handy for jobs in the garden. Cutting big trees is best left to the professional as sudden giving way of the cut end may cause catastrophe. Ensure that children do not eat berries from trees unless these are known to be safe.

The incidence of asthma and hay fever are increasing. These conditions are triggered by allergy and are called atopic diseases. Allergies are now increasing to fruit, nuts, drugs and to latex. Latex is present in rubber gloves. Allergy to latex was almost unknown before 1980, nowadays almost 8% of health workers appear to suffer with this. The increased allergy rate may perhaps be due to cleaner homes and smaller families, leading to less-well developed immune systems. Allergies may also be higher in children born by Caesarean section. Exposure to bacteria and viruses early in life may have an important impact on health. Early exposure to allergens or microorganisms may affect whether or not there is a later development of heart disease, diabetes, cancer and allergies. Asthma and allergy seems to have a reduced incidence in farmers and their families possibly because they are exposed early on in life to many allergens. The message may be to stop using so many disinfectants and cleansers. These agents may have a place but perhaps modern man is overusing them. Another suggestion for the increase in atopic disease is that people who get them may have some alteration in their intestinal microflora. Microflora are bacteria normally present in the gut. Research is ongoing to see if probiotics, which are orally administered micro-organisms, might help these conditions by readjustment of the intestinal microflora. So far there is no convincing evidence that probiotics can prevent or help the symptoms of asthma or hay fever.

Hay fever can lead to unpleasant symptoms with red eyes and nasal stuffiness, due to over-reaction to allergens. Hay fever often begins in the teens but lots of people outgrow it as the immune system matures. Fungal spores may cause symptoms in winter while tree pollens are responsible for at least a quarter of hay fever cases in spring with grass pollen active in summer. Asthma sufferers have more asthmatic attacks during the pollen season. Certain foods (olive oil) and pregnancy can exacerbate hay fever while other foods (eggs, milk, oily fish, yoghurt, wholegrains and vegetables) may improve symptoms. To help symptoms during a high pollen count keep body exposure to a minimum by wearing sunglasses, drying clothes inside, taking a shower after being outside and keeping the car windows shut if possible. Avoid exposure to tobacco smoke, exhaust fumes and perfume which can make the hay fever worse. To ease nasal stuffiness it is helpful to use a bowl of steaming water containing eucalyptus or menthol drops. If all these measures fail to improve symptoms it may be necessary to get a low-dose steroid nasal spray or non-drowsy-forming antihistamine medication.

A new air filter, that removes particles as small as one-millionth of a millimetre from the air, may reduce allergy and hay fever.

People with allergies are more prone than non-allergy sufferers to a condition called keratoconus. This causes the cornea in the eye to become cone-shaped rather than the normal curve. Vision becomes blurred. The condition is usually manifest in the late teens but it can be diagnosed at any age. Glasses or contact lenses may help but a corneal transplant may become necessary.

If walking in a heavily planted area it is wise to keep the skin covered (hat, long trousers and long sleeves) to avoid reactions to plants or insect bites. If bitten, a bee sting should be removed with tweezers taking care not to squeeze the poison into the skin. Generally an anti-inflammatory cream available over the counter is very soothing or apply a solution of 1 teaspoon of sodium bicarbonate (baking powder) in a glass of water. Wasp stings are more likely in the autumn. A wasp retains its sting. An antihistamine cream available over the counter is very soothing but an antihistamine tablet which is not sleep-inducing may be necessary if swelling develops around the area of the bite. One in 200 people will become allergic to bee or wasp stings after being stung. Those who are allergic to bee and wasp venom should carry an adrenaline preparation which is easily administered into any muscle. There are two strengths, for children and adults respectively.

Do not leave swimming pools, wells or expanses of water accessible to young children who may fall into them. Think one step ahead of the child and spot and predict possible dangers. Parents must supervise children in and outside the garden. Children must be warned about the dangers of entering building sites, derelict property or areas with electric pylons. If the child cannot read the danger signs forbidding site entry then the parent must ensure he understands what the signs mean.

Lead pollution can cause serious health issues particularly in children. Parents must be aware of the location of their children at all times and ensure that they themselves do not get involved in the dumping of batteries or other materials likely to cause serious damage to health from environmental pollution. Be a good citizen! Do not do what you yourself would condemn others for doing. Better understanding between travellers and settled people must be encouraged and both groups must be educated to respect the environment by avoiding all types of littering and dumping. Our health and clean air depend on it.

Key sentences: Chemicals released into the sea may be altering the sex of fish, with ovarian tissue being found in the testes of the male fish. If we pollute the fish we pollute ourselves. Parents must supervise children in and outside the garden.

9

In The Workplace

In Ireland the incidence of occupational injuries is high per head of population. In 2004, 49 people lost their lives through workplace injuries. There have been at least 68 work-place deaths in 2005. Most lives were lost in the construction and agriculture sectors with significant contributions from transport and fishing. The most common accident causes overall, included falls from heights, being struck by something collapsing or overturning or contact by moving machine parts. There were 17 deaths on farms in 2005 and 2 of these were children, compared to 13 in 2004. The hazards of tractors have been mentioned many times in the media and in Health and Safety reports. Anyone using a tractor must ensure that adequate training has been obtained to drive carefully, that all safety precautions are observed and that the rules of the road are adhered to. Trailer use must be safe and attention paid to its stability, its connections and its loading. While driving, it is important to avoid sitting on plastic covers or seats for extended periods as a pilonidal cyst may result. Farm and domestic animals need proper supervision and control. The use of luminous neck bands for identification of animals at night should be helpful. Binge drinking has increased in construction site workers. This needs to stop in order to save lives.

Fishing accidents are increasing and attention must be given to sea-worthiness of boats and the ability of fishermen to swim. The Irish Water Safety has emphasized the need to service and check personal and communal flotation devices, such as lifejackets, regularly. Wear and tear at the folds, straps and fastenings should be examined. Gas bottles on inflatable lifejackets should be full, fitted correctly and have no signs of corrosion. Lifejackets should never be used as cushions. The Department of Communications, Marine and Natural Resources and the Irish Coast Guard have produced a booklet regarding lifejacket maintenance and these are available free of charge.

A Work Statement which is essential for managing safely, must be present on all building sites and in workplaces. It is important to listen to and to read instructions before commencing work or using equipment. When accidents occur in the workplace, serious deficiencies may be present in a combination of safety training, understanding of safety documentation, safety equipment and safety officer deployment. Work directives may be totally incomprehensible to some workers because of poor or absent reading ability or language difficulty. All of these issues need to be addressed as a matter of extreme urgency.

Stress is a significant cause of absence from work, replacing back pain as the most commonly cited problem on medical certificates. Stress gives rise to unease, low productivity, increased risk taking leading to accidents, high sickness absence, addictive behaviour and mental health effects including suicide. Alcohol excess may cause or exacerbate stress. Doctors are three times more likely to have cirrhosis and one in 15 may be addicted to drugs or alcohol. Small businesses in Ireland lose about 170 million Euro per year through absenteeism, however there are greater problems with absenteeism in larger businesses. Most absenteeism occurs in the electronics industry followed by the clothing and footwear sectors and the areas worst hit include the Midlands and the North-East. It is thought that in these jobs boredom may arise because of the repetitive nature of the work and in the areas mentioned workers may spend a lot of time travelling to and from work. Better public transport is needed to allow people to come to work in a refreshed state. Further education, training, research and development are important to avoid employees spending long periods of time in boring jobs. While not everything can be computerized or mechanized, repetitive work is often done better by robotic control. There will however always be important jobs that require repetitive human skills and it is important that the need for such work is emphasized by good communication and job allocation, and that appropriate recognition is given to excellence in attendance and to constructive team work. Team work however must not force individual thinking to be submerged by group thinking.

Factors which affect the workforce include:

- age and levels of fitness,

- education, experience, training,

- home conditions including adequate sleep,

- drug or alcohol dependency,

- environmental factors such as good lighting, appropriate temperature, ventilation and meal breaks,

- management which must know its business and must never compromise on safety.

Accidents increase in bad working environments and if the temperature increases over 20° C. More minor accidents occur in the young who are usually more agile but less experienced than the older worker. The older employee may however suffer more severe accidents resulting in a greater degree of disability. It is important to match a worker to his experience and level of fitness. Training must be given with appropriate supervision. We now live in a 24-hr society with supermarkets in a lot of Irish towns open all hours. While there has always been shift work in hospitals, it is now widespread. It is important for all workers to get adequate sleep. Night shifts are somewhat artificial however they are necessary and shift workers must get adequate sleep during the day. There are usually less accidents at night and they are likely to occur after midnight. During the night shift it is important to give adequate breaks for meals and use of toilet facilities. During the break it is essential to walk around and to take an appropriate snack. High protein, low carbohydrate snacks make workers more alert and add less calories. Adequate facilities for the breaks such as a well lit room with a fridge and microwave oven should be supplied. Avoid standing for long periods of time as the column of blood in the veins may exacerbate varicose veins or haemorrhoids (piles).

The EU Signs at Work regulations require that only those signs can be used in relation to the situations they describe. These signs must draw attention rapidly and unambiguously to situations capable of causing hazard. The signs are either prohibition, warning, mandatory or emergency and have specific shapes and colours.

If deep trenches are being dug, never work in them without having appropriate protection on all sides to ensure that no one will be buried alive. If you think that something or some equipment is unsafe it is your right to discuss this with your supervisor. Your rights are protected by law.

Asbestos has friable fibres which must not be disturbed either by physical or inhalational contact. Only those personnel with adequate training to deal with this or other similar material should work with asbestos.

In a garage, naked flames must never be used in close proximity to fuels. Premises must be well-ventilated and particularly so, where fumes are present on a continuous basis.

Air quality can affect those subjects suffering with asthma. Unventilated farm silos where green crops undergo fermentation for use as animal fodder can give off nitrogen oxides which can cause acute or chronic lung disease. Ozone may be formed in and around electrical equipment., in air and water-purifying devices and around printing inks and copying devices which use powerful ultraviolet light sources. It can cause chest pain, persistent cough, sore throat and nosebleeds and dryness of the eyes and throat. Always ensure good ventilation. The permitted levels of all these pollutants are regulated by the EU.

Using ladders by the unskilled DIY person is fraught with danger. Never use a ladder unless the flat surface rests on a solid stable surface. Secure the ladder to the building at the correct angle. Do not stretch or lean. Keep one hand on the ladder. Movement can dislodge the upper part of the ladder and unless such movement is guarded against, it is always desirable that a second person stands at the bottom of the ladder while the other individual climbs to carry out the required task. Special attachments to hold the ladder away from the wall makes access to gutters easier when painting. Accidents with ladders are increasing and often lead to death and serious injury. Even a short fall from a ladder may cause serious damage to the spine, the head or to the extremities. The use of ladders for work purposes may soon be limited. New EU rules may insist for example that where possible windows are cleaned by a long brush reaching from ground to window with a safety platform needed in high-rise buildings.

Electric shock can occur at work. Do not touch the victim if he is in contact with the electric current. Always try to switch off the mains or pull out the plug. Push the victim away from the electric source using a non-metallic object i.e. something wooden like a brush or chair. Large hardboard slabs should never be carried on the head. These may cause pressure not only on the head and neck but also may be a cause of profound soft tissue, tendon and bone injury in the event of slippage. The use of a trolley to which the slab must be properly attached, is appropriate. Recent information has indicated that only 20% of people who sustained burns while at work had first aid services available to them at their workplace. Simple first aid, including cooling down the burnt area by water, could significantly improve the outcome for such subjects.

Eyes and ears are delicate organs. Eye protection must be worn where indicated. There is nothing more foolish than road-workers without goggles who pound away at concrete without realizing the potential risk of serious eye damage. Many people work in environments where noise is constant such as building sites and factory floors. Excessive noise in the workplace results in long-term damage to a significant proportion of the workforce. Noise can be a problem in the entertainment and music industry but any work area can cause problems. In addition to hearing loss, noise at work can contribute to accidents, work-related stress and general ill-health. Although noise has been officially recognized as the major preventable cause of deafness, attitudes to ear protection are still half-hearted.

Ears must be protected against excessive noise. In the workplace, the appropriate work-gear provided must be worn i.e. use of ear muffs, goggles and protective clothing. Never say "I do not need this". You do! There are two main types of ear protector, those based on the ear plug, and the headset which is hygienic and lasts a long time. The headset also warns co-workers that communication may require a little extra effort. While wearing ear protectors it is important that the person is made aware of any traffic in the vicinity as the noise of an approaching vehicle may be considerably diminished. Sustained noise can also cause a problem called tinnitus. This may be felt merely as an annoying sensation or at the other extreme, as the sound of a jet engine. There is apparently a strong link between emotion and the level of tinnitus and relaxation has a role to play in treatment. A new EU Directive will be put in place in the near future which will set a limit of 87 decibels for workers' daily exposure to noise.

Some primary school teachers in Ireland have cited problems with chronic hoarseness and laryngitis from using their voices loudly all day long in order to control children in the classroom. With the huge problems with illiteracy it is appropriate to address discipline at home and at school and measures taken to enforce this. It is also worth remembering that rowdy undisciplined schoolchildren can become much more manageable if they consume a healthy diet. New research has shown that when fast food such as hot dogs and chips was changed to boiled beef, vegetable and potato with water or apple juice replacing sugary drinks, the concentration and energy of children improved substantially. It is time for teachers and parents to act together to address this issue.

Epilepsy can sometimes be manifest at work. The employee may not have mentioned this during the pre-work medical examination or may not have had the condition at that time. Seizures lasting several minutes can be triggered by stress, excess alcohol or rarely by flickering lights. Protect the head. Do not put anything in the mouth. Once the seizure is over, ensure that the person is on his side in the recovery position to avoid inhalation of stomach contents. Subjects with prolonged seizures must be sent to hospital. Appropriate but understanding discussion between the person involved and his employer should ensure that he is not a danger to himself or others. Employment away from operating machinery should be offered as appropriate.

Management must set example by wearing all appropriate safety gear such as clothing, ear defenders, helmet and goggles. All must be aware of the law with regard to safety, noise and substances such as lead and asbestos. All relevant companies should have an adequate and practical rapid response to accidents and chemical incidents. The responsibility of the site, office or hospital manager is to ensure that appropriate advice has been taken and is being followed. The safety and well-being of all fellow workers depend on good management.

Every employer should have appropriately trained first aid personnel on each shift. Training should be from an expert who should review and update training procedures on a regular basis. All emergency numbers must be listed on a notice-board. Proficiency in resuscitation is useful. This should be acquired at an appropriate accredited centre and it is also taught in some workplaces. In the US special easy-to-use equipment for restoration of heart rhythm is available at designated sites for use by lay people with expertise in its use. Similar equipment is available at a few designated Irish centres. In time this practice may become more widespread as more user-friendly equipment becomes available.

During your working day be it manual work or office work be as comfortable as possible. Do the work well but use all available opportunity to avoid unnecessary strain or danger. Working excessive hours is not a good idea as it will lead to stress at home and at work. No one is indispensable and everyone can be replaced. Even if you are the boss, set aside leisure hours. Missing out on family occasions can cause tension, excess road speed and danger to your own life and those of others.

New health and safety legislation, due to come into force in early 2006, makes provision for future regulations seeking to prevent deaths and injuries in the workplace by testing individuals for intoxicants. While fears have been expressed that this procedure might infringe civil rights, certain transport companies already test their staff randomly for alcohol and drug use and have obtained a 100% compliance rate. The common good must prevail in order to reduce RTAs and other accidents due to alcohol and drugs. A pilot who recently landed his plane too fast admitted to suffering from physiological and psychological fatigue at the time of the landing. His mental trauma was apparently due to marital problems. These problems had affected his ability to eat and sleep normally. Human error can prove costly so it is appropriate for management to be alert to human frailty and to unease for whatever reason, amongst staff. Human resource departments often fall short of help for all its staff and may be inclined to use clichés learnt from psychology books rather than actually giving meaningful support.

Irish workers in general appear to travel from commuter towns in quite large numbers. Hopefully with the recent announcement that Ireland's transport system is to get a cash boost, better public transport systems will enable many workers to leave their cars at home. The commuter towns should also be given public libraries with computer facilities in order to reduce anti-social behaviour largely due to lack of educational facilities. No one however must be allowed to vandalize public facilities including toilets, libraries or buses. Provincial schools need to be upgraded with avoidance of 'best school' segregation to a few major cities.

A recent survey has revealed that contrary to some beliefs, Irish bosses do not have to spend much time commuting to work. Almost 70% spend less than an hour travelling to and from work and 9% are able to walk to work. However, 40% of business owners in Ireland are suffering from stress due to a combination of demanding customers, increased competition and pressure on profit margins, lack of time with family and 'red tape'. In comparison with these stresses, keeping up with innovation is not a big factor. It is a delusion to think that one is indispensable. If you can afford it get an assistant or partner, settle for less profit but better quality of life. By planning, management, accepting smaller profit margins and delegation, work stress can be minimized. The Asian countries are hugely stressed (50-70%) while Sweden is the low-stress country of the business world.

Manual healthcare workers are more at risk of ill-health on retirement than non-manual workers, with muscle and bone disorders, mental illness and circulatory disorders accounting for most illnesses. Repetitive manual work over an extended period of time can lead to boredom, and negative attitudes. It is imperative that continued education and re-training be offered to all manual workers in an effort to limit the periods spent in such posts. Skills need to undergo continuous upgrading throughout one's working life. Literacy must be improved in order for workers to advance their career opportunities.

Although there is no definitive evidence that mobile phones are dangerous to health, avoid over-use of a mobile phone. In a rural area the signal is more intense because of the location of cables so it is important to use the mobile prudently.

For the health and welfare of all our citizens, population, jobs and good educational facilities need to be spread around the country and a sustainable rural economy established.

Key sentences: Accidents increase in bad working environments and if the temperature increases over 20° C. The responsibility of the site, office or hospital manager is to ensure that appropriate advice has been taken and is being followed. The safety and well being of all fellow workers depend on good management.

10

On The Road

A recent EU survey has shown that Ireland is one of only three countries in western Europe where the number of road deaths rose in 2004. The number of deaths rose by 13% to 379. Of the 19 countries surveyed, Ireland had the biggest increase followed by Turkey and Greece. In 2005 the situation got even worse and there were 399 deaths due to road traffic accidents (RTAs) in the Republic of Ireland, the highest figure since 2001 when 411 deaths occurred on the road. The number of people arrested for drink-driving during the 2005 Christmas holiday season increased by 14% compared to 2004. By contrast, the road deaths in Northern Ireland in 2005 were the lowest for several decades in spite of a substantial increase in car ownership, and drink-driving arrests increased by 4% compared to 2004.

The 'international norm' for RTAs which is based on population, indicates that approximately 20 deaths per month might occur in the Republic of Ireland. However currently there is more than one death per day leading to at least 150 deaths per year more than expected by international standards. There are also approximately 1,200 serious injuries more than expected for our population which means rehabilitation beds are occupied for indefinite periods of time. People are left with serious debilitating injuries from which they may never fully recover. Traffic congestion has reached high levels which could be avoided by appropriate infrastructure and a good public transport system. By the time the congestion is reduced much damage will needlessly be caused to the environment and many more injuries will occur on the roads and in our cities.

The number of needless deaths and road injuries tends in general to be higher the less sophisticated the country and its inhabitants. Good discipline and sophistication go together. An 'all-round' educated, healthy and established society tends to care for its fellow citizens by having a good public transport system, appropriate Health and Safety at Work and road rules that in general are followed and treated with respect. In a recent survey which examined seat belt use, speeding and drink-driving, Ireland ranked 13 out of 25 EU countries and fared badly on drink-driving and enforcement of traffic laws. Finland, Sweden, the UK, Germany and the Netherlands fared well in these areas and all have lower RTAs than Ireland. Portugal, Spain Latvia, Poland, Estonia and Lithuania were all like Ireland in the lower half of the table. During the first four months of 2006 the death toll on Irish roads is the worst since 2000.

86% of RTAs are due to human error. Far too many deaths and injuries are caused by excessive speed, drug and alcohol abuse, negligent driving and tiredness at the wheel or suicidal intention. Young men drive too fast on roads not designed for speed. Men aged 17-24 years account for 6% of the population but 1 in 5 driver deaths. Attention deficit hyperactivity disorder (ADHD) may be a factor in RTAs although poor discipline at home and at school may be just as likely to have caused negligent and dangerous driving. ADHD is commoner in males and in offspring of women who have consumed alcohol during pregnancy. With the significant illiteracy rate in Ireland and the variable level of comprehension of the rules of the road, it is worrying to think that some drivers cannot read or may not fully understand road signs. In 2004, 24 pedestrians were killed on Irish roads. In the first few months of 2006 at least 8 pedestrians have lost their lives. Many of these have been killed through no fault of their own by careless drivers, however some pedestrians seem to have little awareness of moving traffic. In cities, people who walk in front of moving traffic tend to be careless or lack insight, however a proportion may be physically or mentally unwell and these must be helped and cared for too.

All drivers must be made aware of the huge burden of road accidents and deaths on relatives, on A & E and on the people left with a life of permanent disability caused by excessive road speed and drink-driving. While all accidents may not be preventable, every effort must be put in place to reduce injuries on the road. Accident prevention demands continual education. People need educating that preventing accidents is their personal responsibility. Since so many young people are involved in RTAs, education about the rules of the road and the responsibilities of pedestrians and drivers must be taught from an early age. The first step is to educate the pedestrian about rules of the road. This must be taught by parents and reinforced at primary school.

The penalty points system for drivers needs strict enforcement with high financial and licence endorsement penalties for offenders. Speed limits should be sensible and therefore more likely to be observed. No one is too busy to adhere to speed limits. A driver who has been found speeding on more than one occasion should in addition to monetary and driving licence penalties, be made to take a refresher course in sensible driving with emphasis on driving within the speed limit and without alcohol. A legal system that allows drivers who have breached the law to get away with technicalities must be immediately reviewed. Driving tests must be adequate to examine a potential driver in the driving conditions prevailing in 2006. Proficiency in the rules of the road must be achieved. No 'provisional licence' drivers should be allowed unaccompanied on the road. The wearing of seat belts must be enforced and the message **'Never drink and drive'** continually reinforced at home, at school and in pubs. Motor bike drivers must observe all rules aimed particularly at them. Servicing of public and private vehicles must be done to an acceptably high international standard. Trailers on vehicles must be adequately regulated. Hand-held mobile phones must not be used while driving. Bicyclists must be responsible and take adequate safety precautions and be seen.

Dual carriageways are associated with a lower number of traffic accidents. In Ireland there are not enough dual carriageways so extra vigilance and attention to road signs, with prohibition of overtaking on narrow roads, are needed. Overtaking in a left- hand drive car is more hazardous than usual so consideration must be given as to whether such vehicles should be allowed on our roads. There is controversy whether or not CCTV cameras reduce accidents. In the UK almost 1 in 3 car crashes happens within a mile of the driver's home. On familiar routes the driver tends to switch off. Strategic cameras should be adequate for dual carriageway observation however they are unlikely to pick up a drunk driver driving erratically but still within the speed limit. CCTV cameras are useful at traffic lights in order to spot those drivers who drive through red lights risking death to pedestrians and other motorists. The cameras are not an adequate replacement for garda patrols which should be deployed in order to allow a concentrated clamp-down on drink-driving, speeding and careless driving. Gardaí on patrol are the best deterrent and there is a need for more of them particularly in those counties with a particularly bad record for road deaths such as Donegal, Louth, Dublin and Cork. Smaller narrow country roads should be patrolled regularly. The National Safety Council (NSC) has stressed the need for random testing for both drugs and alcohol. These tests must be robust and legally acceptable. Gardaí must be adequately trained in the use of roadside and station breathalysers. A garda presence at busy traffic lights is always reassuring but may not always be feasible. Traffic lights should be patrolled by a traffic warden until care in crossing has been taught and reinforced.

New traffic headlamps that reduce glare for oncoming traffic and adapt to corners, road and weather conditions should be available in the future. Driver inattention often causes accidents. Inbuilt radar may be able to detect if the driver's car is getting too close to the car in front. Multisensory non-visual signals may promote rapid response in order to avoid accidents. Vibrating seatbelts, imaginary car horns and citrus scents could soon be important car safety devices. These warning systems could reduce the number of front-to-rear collisions however it will be some time before cars can be fitted with technology capable of overcoming human error.

There is no reason to think that subjects with epilepsy, high blood pressure cardiac problems or diabetic patients taking insulin, make a substantial contribution to RTAs. As for all road users however, subjects taking tablets or injections must be conversant with the medical aspects of fitness to drive for their own sake and for public safety. Individual responses must be considered by doctors when advising controlled epileptic patients who are applying for driving licences. Hypoglycaemia (low blood sugar) may impair tracking ability in diabetic patients and the subject may be unaware of the impairment. If you are taking any tablets or injections it is important to be stabilized on these before driving. Your general practitioner will advise you regarding this and also what you must declare regarding your eyesight and health when applying for a driving licence. Pharmacists should label with particular emphasis any medicine likely to affect driving.

First aid is the ability to perform the essential emergency treatment of an injury in order to help the injured party. It is important first of all, not to further injure the subject with inappropriate intervention. Proficiency in resuscitation is useful. This should be acquired at an appropriate accredited centre and is also taught in some workplaces. If substantial blood or fluid loss has been sustained, jeans should not be removed from the victim until fluid replacement has been started since the jeans act like the US military anti-shock trousers. Cardio-pulmonary resuscitation can keep the brain and heart supplied with blood and oxygen until medical help arrives. In the US special easy-to-use equipment for restoration of heart rhythm is available at designated sites for use by lay people with expertise in its use. Similar equipment is available at a few designated Irish centres including sports venues. In time this practice may become more widespread as more user-friendly equipment becomes available.

In spite of the large numbers of head injuries relative to our population such injuries cannot be treated in small local A&E departments. With the suggested reforms of the Irish Health Services it is likely that the percentage of the population reaching an adequately resourced A & E department within one hour following an RTA would actually fall by approximately 10%. Treatment within one hour is vital as the 'golden hour' is the period when treatment is likely to produce the best outcome. An expert report has suggested that relocation of ambulance services might be necessary, with ambulances being based at designated locations in communities rather than at ambulance bases. In response to this suggestion there are now plans for rapid response ambulance services for the Mid-West. The proposed reforms will need an overall review particularly given our huge RTA rate, but accident prevention must remain the major goal.

Counselling for bereaved families, relatives and acquaintances has become a regular feature in recent years. This is obviously a very last resort. Resources must be concentrated on accident prevention.

Key sentence: All drivers must be made aware of the huge burden of road accidents and deaths on relatives, on A & E and on the people left with a life of permanent disability caused by excessive road speed and drink-driving.

11

Growing Up

Children must be nurtured. Life today is stressful and excessive stress is the main hindrance to our enjoyment of life. Young people are experiencing more social and psychological problems than ever before and at an earlier age. Parents have a huge responsibility to ensure that their children grow up with guidance and a responsible attitude both to themselves, towards others and towards the environment. A balance must be sought between school, home and social lives. Excess structured activities is tiring for both parents and children. Parents worry that playgrounds may be a magnet for drug addicts and sellers of drugs. There must therefore be safe places for children to play and playing fields where children can work off excess energy without resorting to vandalism. In the UK the government plans to make state-sponsored 'parenting' classes available because there are fears that present-day parenting is not as good as in previous generations. The majority of parents probably know what must be done although many feel inhibited from showing adequate discipline. The so-called 'pushover parents' either indulge their children or leave them to 'find their own way'. Parents therefore if necessary should seek guidance themselves to ensure that their children have the best possible advice for work and play and for consequent mental and physical growth. The young must have stability and a sense of being valued. They must learn to respect their parents. Children should not be physically or verbally abused. Both tend to make children aggressive and lead to low emotional intelligence.

It is important to ensure that the child does not grow up too soon without the full experience of childhood. Parent power should not be allowed to undermine school discipline.

Good health and effective education go together. The intelligence quotient (IQ) is affected by a child's environmental stimulation. Long-term exposure to air pollution affects lung function in children and teenagers and causes absence from school. There is evidence that children who are dehydrated (not enough water to drink) are slower at arithmetic and prone to tiredness. While inadequate water should not be a problem in Ireland lack of adequate nutrition which can occur through poverty or ignorance will affect concentration and physical and mental development. Priorities often get muddled, with huge pressure being put on families mainly by the children themselves, to make an expensive social occasion out of school or religious events. Around one million Euro was paid out from social services to assist with expenses for these events in 2004. The cost of dresses, hairdressers, photographers and beauty salons contributed to the parents' need for social assistance. With all this spending on fashion there may be little money left for essentials. The purpose of the event is often lost when fashion competition takes over. Priorities must be established and parents must not be responsible for pushing children into adulthood too early by dressing female children especially, in adult fashion.

While children of mothers who go out to work do not have a worse school record than children of mothers who work in the home, surveys reveal that what most parents and children want is to spend as much time as possible together. Often however economic need or perceived need may push mothers into the workplace. Young children may or may not develop better socially and emotionally if they are looked after by their mothers compared to nannies, child-minders or grandparents. Women who enjoy working outside the home should be under no pressure to give this up but adequate provision must be made for child care. Most women who work part-time seem to be able to cope with home and work and this type of arrangement should be encouraged by employers. What is most important is to create a stable environment for children rather than somewhere to leave them when parents go out to work.

There is some evidence to show that children who are in nursery care for long hours at the beginning of their first year of life are more aggressive and disobedient than other children. However a recent research study has also shown that children who attended day care centres in the first six months of life had a lower risk of childhood leukaemia. The timing and pattern of infections is important and contact with other children during nursery care may lead to exposure to non-serious infection and better development of the immune system. It is thought that a poorly developed immune system arising out of lack of early exposure to common infections, might allow cancer cells to develop following infection in those who are genetically susceptible to cancer. Therefore while nursery care was previously thought to be most beneficial after the age of two it might also be beneficial in the first year of life provided the child is not away from home for long periods. It is also desirable that nursery care in the first year of life has a high minder to baby ratio and that the same minder sees the same infants on a regular basis. Attention to the child's sleep requirements is important regardless of who minds the child. Five month old children have been found to have bigger attention span if they sleep for long periods during the day. The wise course seems to be that an early bed-time and good day-time naps are beneficial.

The future generation must be protected from illiteracy, promiscuity, alcohol and drug abuse

Children with poor self-esteem may get involved with people and situations that are not good for them and will put up with behaviour from their peers which is unacceptable. Sadly such children may take drugs and alcohol just to be accepted. They compromise their integrity just to be liked. Children must be encouraged to bring their friends home. At least parents will know where and with whom they are spending their leisure hours. Possible involvement in alcohol or drug taking must be investigated and strongly discouraged. Advice in handling such an event may have to be sought. Juvenile delinquency is often associated with poor parenting. Boredom and lack of skills are often present. Children at-risk may have frequent illnesses or learning difficulties. Sometimes hearing or visual disorders or coordination problems may be present. The feeling of inadequacy needs to be removed in order to give the child an aim in life. Parents and teachers should boost the child's self-esteem where possible. People with high self-esteem are happier, are less likely to be depressed and tend to be more persistent in achieving a goal than those with low self-esteem. Every child must be encouraged to use whatever ability he has by learning new skills in or outside the family group. The GP can be very helpful by coordinating any specific medical service required to treat the physical deficiencies.

It is important to ensure that Attention Deficit Hyperactivity Disorder (ADHD) is not missed as this may present as delinquency. ADHD may cause a child to underachieve academically and to cause trouble and tension in and around the family and school environment, in spite of having received good parenting. ADHD is usually a hereditary condition with a close male relative often found to be affected by the same problem. Alcohol taken in pregnancy has also been associated with ADHD in the child. Many children with ADHD although immature both socially and emotionally are often intellectually advanced but find it hard to complete their work unless directly supervised. Correct diagnosis is important in order to allow the subject to attain their full potential. Treatment includes behavioural therapy, avoiding confrontation, boosting of achievement and if necessary the appropriate use of stimulant medication.

Parents can teach their children to ask questions, to evaluate situations and choices, to be kind and not to bully the shy individual. Girls can be more divisive and skilled at bullying than boys so care must be taken to ensure that your child is not a bully and is also protected from this type of behaviour. Children like adults need to be aware that there is no such thing as a free lunch and that drug taking or selling, or indulgence in alcohol excess may kill them or scar them for life. Respect for animals and the environment must be taught at home and at school. Parents must teach their children that cruelty to animals can never be tolerated. There is evidence that cruelty to animals can lead to cruelty and assault on humans.

Parents must not allow their children to eat excessively and thereby become obese because fat cells deposited and enlarged in childhood may lead to physical and social problems in adulthood. Childhood obesity increases the risk for diabetes and heart disease, and already cases of heart disease are being seen in Irish teenagers. Obesity in early life is linked to a risk of hospitalization and death from heart disease when older. As the 'fat kid' at school the child will appear grotesque with a big stomach and a neck lost in flab and may be the focus of bullying, leading to loss of self esteem. Mothers can influence their children's tastes in food. Research has indicated that the flavors experienced in the first four months after birth are critical in determining a child's subsequent tastes. Flavours from the food eaten by a woman while breast feeding percolate into breast milk giving her children a potentially lifelong taste for similar foods. The baby is exposed to the flavours that the mother eats. What the mother eats is accepted as being safe. Children may like the food that their mothers ate for the rest of their lives so sensible eating by the mother is important. Parents must however avoid obsession with diet or get fixations on healthy eating. Eating disorders may occur as a result of this obsession. **The aim must be to eat sensibly, have occasional treats but avoid extremes in anything.**

In spite of a lot of criticism, school dinners are better than lunchboxes filled with crisps, fizzy drinks and cereal bars The school lunchbox should contain a bottle of milk or water (plain or flavoured) and a child-approved nutritious lunch. The latter should contain the sensible foods already discussed with a combination of meat, vegetable, fruit and wholegrain bread. Sensible food can be made both appetizing and nutritious. Go easy on the salt and add some pepper or herbs. Some food companies have launched a food labelling initiative aimed at 13-15 year olds which should be quite understandable by this age group. While sweets, crisps, biscuits or chocolate can be eaten occasionally, all four should be avoided on a regular basis to avoid obesity and dental caries.

If a child becomes obese it is essential to loose the excess weight as soon as possible. Research in the 8-12 year-old group has shown that for successful weight reduction parental involvement is critical. What appears vitally important is an overall and consistent change in lifestyle and diet of the whole family, emphasizing that while on occasions adherence to a good diet might lapse, the essential objective is to ensure that for the most part, a prudent diet is combined with some form of exercise. Daily walks including to school and back if this is practical is ideal but any form of exercise which is safe is acceptable. Bicycles unfortunately increase child injuries so supervision and good bicycle training is mandatory. A sensible weight-achieving approach should be adopted. Machines selling chocolate bars and other snacks are not a good idea in schools and if present, children should only have access to these once weekly. The entire school community approach must be harnessed and all encouraged to achieve better overall health and education.

Eating disorders appear to be levelling out in Europe and in the US. Early identification is necessary because early treatment is associated with improved outcome. In the long-term, television has responsibility to ensure that children's programmes do not project abnormal thinness as being the 'norm'. It seems that the Barbie doll image is not too popular any more but what will replace this? The ideal female form must be portrayed as a composite of adequate proportions ruled by a healthy enquiring mind rather than placing disproportionate emphasis on appearance.

Advice should be given to the teenager as early as this can be understood, in order to try to avoid many of today's potential pitfalls including drugs, alcohol and sexual promiscuity. In many schools it has been reported that Monday seems to be a 'hangover' day with many students a million miles away. There is also a tendency for truculence with fewer students amenable to correction. A recent survey has shown that Irish students spend 80 million Euro on drink per year and that the majority enjoy binge drinking. 40% admitted to using cannabis, and ecstasy was the second most-used illegal drug. Sexual disease prevalence is now high in Ireland with sexual intercourse occurring in teenagers. This can affect both sexual reproduction and the general health with serious consequences. Untreated sexual disease can lead to sterility particularly in females and to general disease including death from immunosuppression. 'Binge smoking' (which is a prolonged use over a short time) of cannabis can lead to fatal strokes. 'Binge smoking' has recently left one teenager with paralysis and two others dead. Unfortunately there is a common belief that cannabis is less dangerous than other recreational drugs. It is essential to realize that cannabis is a dangerous drug that can cause abnormal physical and mental states from which subjects may never recover.

Children often criticize their parents. Sometimes they feel that this is something that has to be done in order to project a 'cool' independent attitude. However in reality, each child or young adult wants their parents to look after them and help to get them started in life. School and learning should be a happy experience where there is interaction and motivation. Learning is achieved by an individual who is not worried by internal or external events and is made to feel unique, creative and successful. Young people look for comfort when upset but sometimes there are issues which they will not share even with their closest friends. Interaction at home and at school is very important at this time to avoid small but important issues becoming major problems. Teachers and parents must give adequate support even if this means that parents have to go back to school themselves! Parents can help most by liaison with school to ensure that their child is coping with any undue stress, has adequate well-being with acceptable self-esteem and no major problems involving academic performance. If there is a problem in any of these areas the school should advise the parents and children regarding coping strategies. Parents must avoid nagging but remain in charge and become expert at negotiation. Avoid conflict. Give time for discussion. Allow children to say anything on their mind. Parents must get across to children that they care about whatever the topic happens to be. They must also show that they believe in something which they want to communicate to their children. Discipline is important and must be mutually discussed and accepted.

It is frightening to realize that more than 10% of Irish people are illiterate with many more at the lowest level of literacy. Poor education and poor health go hand in hand. It has been known for decades that disease is frequently higher in the lower socio-economic groups and poor people die younger than their socially advantaged contemporaries. A recent report of a survey in 12 primary schools in disadvantaged areas has revealed that 50% have low reading scores, 75% have a very poor knowledge of mathematics with fifth and sixth class pupils being particularly bad. The attendance record is also poor. There is no mention that these children are mentally handicapped. This report reflects badly on teachers as well as parents. In disadvantaged areas, a lower pupil to teacher ratio with early intervention to improve school attendance is necessary if the next generation wants to improve their educational prospects and rise out of their present circumstances.

Children handicapped by lack of basic education are traumatized for life. Education must be about teaching reading, writing and counting and then encouraging each individual to gain some form of qualification. Schools in Ireland have often placed too much emphasis on passing exams. Practical skills are not adequately encouraged in those who excel in these areas. In primary school, children are given little time or encouragement to prepare for the job market. Consequently a lot of teenagers leave school with no confidence, a sense of inadequacy and a feeling of 'no future'. Although a Social Personal Health Education subject is now being taught at Junior Certificate level, it is important that intervention programmes be established in primary schools to help students to deal with everyday stress, to develop social skills and prepare for a career or further education. There should be advice about coping skills with a division between work time and leisure time. Work time should be focused on the aim of study whether this is domestic economy, carpentry, plumbing, computers, or proceeding to further education. Each student should be encouraged to have a hobby, to be a good citizen and to be healthy. Basic advice regarding diet, sleep and general well-being should be available. The primary school teacher's aim must be to ensure by all means possible that the child matures into a self- sufficient adult who can read, write and manage money. If these three basic accomplishments are present, social skills will follow. Emphasis should not be on money but on a means to achieve a happy fulfilled life with a sense of being valued which only individuality can give.

Leisure time should be for relaxation. In Ireland leisure time is often synonymous with alcohol excess. Alcohol consumption as a stress de-fuser must be discouraged as it is a crutch leaned too heavily upon, a source of much of our ill health and garrulousness rather than wit. While some nations may humour us regarding our alcohol consumption, most nations secretly think that we might do a lot better if we could party with less alcohol.

In France where the illiteracy rate is lower than in Ireland special 'boot camps' are being set up by the French army to help school 'dropouts'. The fear that these subjects will be socially excluded for life has prompted the setting up of establishments where participation is voluntary, discipline is tight, dress code is obligatory and respect for authority is demanded. In return social skills are learned and each individual can acquire a qualification that can lead to employment. In Belfast an 'alternative school' gives 'dropout pupils' a second chance. The focus is on taking responsibility for one's life. The project involves a mix of academic and vocational subjects along with personal, social and health education and outdoor hobbies including mountaineering. This seems to be successful however another scheme in the UK which allows youngsters to learn a trade while still at school, has been discredited because of truancy. The UK system may have run into problems because it is not easy to move between sites and adhere to timetables. The French model seems like a better idea and may be followed in other countries.

World-wide there is a substantial rise in the onset of depression at puberty. Puberty is the stage of sexual maturity. The WHO ranks depression as a major cause of disability. Women of child-bearing age who are depressed, may transmit a substantially higher risk of depression to their offspring. Ireland today has a very high suicide rate particularly amongst young men. The reason for this is not entirely clear but certain factors may be contributory. Stress and lifestyle may be factors. Depression is increasing too amongst pets with 8 out of 10 vets reporting an increase in depression-related illnesses amongst their patients. It is thought that the lifestyle of today's pet owners may be to blame with owners leaving pets for a long boring time on their own, without even the radio for company! Perhaps parents are unwittingly doing the same to children. Diabetes is also increasing in dogs possibly because we are too busy or too fat to walk them.

All children feel sad sometimes. It is important to have a good talk with them and to let them talk through their problems. Do not rush into getting them medication for depression. Taking anti-depressants may actually increase the risk of suicide in adolescents. If symptoms are prolonged or if there are signs of unusual behaviour, treatment including medication will be needed. According to research carried out by Irish psychiatrists 1 out of every 3 students who live alone becomes depressed. The average rate of depression amongst college students is 7.8% with this figure apparently rising to 34% in those aged 17-21 years who live alone. The study also found that 15% of those living in campus

100

accommodation experience depression. Alcohol may have a major role in depression and Irish students drink too much because nobody has told them otherwise. Society needs to change fast if the next generation is to rise out of the drunken image stereotype projecting enjoyment, since the majority of those who drink to excess are anything but happy.

Suicide is often highest after Christmas when the festive activities have stopped and a return to normal living is expected. Signs of depression include guilt regarding family problems, aggression, impulsive behaviour, feelings of worthlessness, talk about death and experimenting with drugs or alcohol. A recent study in the UK suggests that suicide rates could be cut by better services for young people with mental illness who also abuse alcohol or drugs and by better treatment of those with depression. Emphasis needs to be put on a more varied lifestyle with an adequate motivation for both work and leisure pursuits. Suicide rates in the UK particularly amongst young men have shown a significant drop in recent years. Research findings in the US have shown that an enzyme, which is a protein which influences chemical processes in the body, called protein kinase C has been linked with mood disorders. This enzyme appears to be significantly less plentiful in those teenagers who committed suicide. This identification may lead to better drug treatment.

Prevention is better than cure. It is important to realize that among mentally disturbed patients, suicide may be 'contagious by imitation' and this may be a situation where preventive measures may be used. Above all, children need to talk about any problems and to get involved in self-development programmes. They must be encouraged to get involved in hobbies or sports. The teenager must find an identity in adolescence. This is difficult because of sexual development and peer pressure. Young people are maturing sexually at an earlier age. Feelings of inadequacy may arise when a slow developer is confronted by peers who have already matured sexually. Along with examination stress there is stress to achieve a job on leaving school or university. There is an added stress of trying to be 'macho' and being able to 'date'. Parents and teachers must be understanding and supportive but strict. Children need to respect themselves, their parents and what they have. Parents must let children know that they can ask for help at any time and advise them if their attitude is wrong. Smoking and excessive alcohol consumption must be discouraged from an early age. Children or teenagers must never be allowed to abuse animals.

Screen violence can harm even well-behaved children. Research has shown that teenagers can suffer from loss of control and from poor decision-making after exposure to violent images. Brain scans have shown reduced activity in the frontal cortex, which is responsible for decision making and self control, in normal subjects exposed to violence. The images were indistinguishable from scans of subjects suffering with disruptive behaviour disorders. While it is debatable how much influence advertisements for food have on children and young adults, it is well known that workers chronically exposed to traumatic or barbaric events such as accidents, violence, war casualties etc, experience considerable psychological aftershock. In the US and the UK measures are being taken to condemn the glorification of guns and knives either in magazines or on the TV. For each hour of TV watched per day a child may gain up to 14 pounds in weight per year because of the crisps, biscuits and fizzy drinks consumed during this time. Studies have found that teenagers who watch lots of sex on TV are more likely to engage in sex compared to teenagers who do not watch such programmes. Online poker is hooking countless young people. Parents should assume responsibility for what the child or teenager is viewing. Video violence is something that can be monitored and screened. A visit to the library or art gallery or to the soccer pitch might be a useful diversion to avoid TV and food obsession. An arrangement to substitute fruit occasionally for fizzy drinks or crisps may make the difference between health and obesity, with risk of diabetes and heart disease in early adulthood.

Mobile phone use may not be healthy for children since the radiation involved is significant and the brain is not fully formed until at least 18 years of age and sometimes does not completely mature until 25 years. Parents need to establish rules for the use of mobile phones. While allowing a certain amount of local calls, permission to use the mobile for overseas calls must be obtained and an arrangement made with the teenager to contribute payment for these. Pocket money allowance must not be extravagant.

Parents must be good role models. Parents' attitudes to people, animals, food, drugs, alcohol, smoking and the environment affect children more than any advertisement or lectures. Parents must be tolerant and show flexibility but keep discipline. Parents must encourage assertiveness but not aggression. Parents must emphasize the dangers of alcohol, drug abuse and early sex. Parents must encourage children to share some household duties, get hobbies and thus avoid boredom and situations leading to harmful physical or mental experience. Overuse of the internet by everyone should be avoided.

Recurrent respiratory infections and cough are the main cause of medical consultations in children. Vaccination against childhood illnesses is therefore necessary . It is also important for parents to avoid smoking and to advise children not to begin to smoke.

15% of children in Ireland have *asthma* and in excess of 20% of school-going children have symptoms consistent with asthma. Asthma probably 'runs' in families but is exacerbated by air pollution, house dust, smoking and certain foods. Living in damp lead- polluted conditions lowers resistance to disease and leads to childhood wheezing. Smoking can trigger previously undiagnosed asthma. It is estimated that in Ireland up to 20% of teenagers between 15 and 18 years take up smoking. Good housing conditions and avoidance of smoking and dumping in the environment can reduce the incidence of asthma and must be the aim of parents or guardians. Demonstration of the damage which smoking can do to the lungs, the heart, the brain and the feet, with illustrative pictures for emphasis, must be part of primary school education. The treatment of asthma includes avoiding any factors that can exacerbate the condition, the appropriate use of medicine (inhalers) for relieving symptoms and the use of other types of medication (inhalers) for preventing asthmatic attacks. Parents, teachers and child-minders must know how to cope in an acute asthmatic emergency. Appropriate use of medication is very important for safe asthma management as it allows one to stay active with more symptom-free days and less need for emergency medication. If you are unsure whether or not your child has asthma, talk to your GP. A booklet is available from The Asthma Society of Ireland. Allergy to peanuts is fairly common in childhood and can occur in association with asthma. It is recommended that children less than 6 years should not eat peanuts.

Children who are obese may respond less well to asthma medication. Subjects with 'difficult to treat asthma' are however generally either not taking the prescribed medication or are suffering from a condition other than asthma. All teenagers with 'non-responsive asthma' should be tested for a genetic condition called alpha-1 antitrypsin (AAT) deficiency which can lead to a serious liver or lung disease. Approximately 1200 people in Ireland have this condition but often it goes undetected and adults may present with chronic cough and disability from emphysema, a disabling lung condition. There is presently no cure for AAT deficiency apart from transplantation. Early detection is important to ensure that the condition is managed appropriately and in particular that the subject avoids smoking and chooses suitable employment which would not exacerbate the condition.

Autism is a developmental disability affecting a person's social and communication skills. Autism is not just one disease but a whole spectrum of conditions often showing withdrawal and a lack of ability to communicate. A brain circuit that helps people to observe and imitate the emotions of others is almost completely switched off in children with autism. It is recognized by impaired development in children often before the age of 3 years. It often occurs, possibly coincidentally, around the time of childhood vaccinations. Autism is known to occur in certain families and to have a genetic biological basis. The autistic individual often shows lack of emotion and of social interaction. These individuals are not able to communicate adequately, are not good at play and their thinking lacks imagination and creativity with a tendency to impose rigid routines on many aspects of day-to-day living. Autistic individuals may show signs of other problems such as fear or phobias, sleeping and eating disturbances, temper tantrums and aggression. Lack of social interaction persists into adult life. Asperger 's syndrome is a high-functioning form of autism. Children with autism can be misdiagnosed as being deaf. It is important that autism is recognized in its various forms in order for the individual to receive the most appropriate education and follow-up. Most individuals with autism respond well to highly structured, specialized programmes and many make enormous contribution to society. An autistic professor in the US has developed a practical system of dealing with animals which helps their management while avoiding unnecessary and thoughtless trauma to them. In a UK study, children with autism who received an intensive form of education in the home showed significant improvement in IQ levels. The GP will offer advice about the various options available.

The education of children who are *deaf* either from birth or before they have learnt to speak can be a challenge. Subjects with congenital deafness should be recognised by at least one year of age. Improvement in early detection of deafness, with the fitting of appropriate high-powered hearing aids have improved the situation however there are some children who will not be able to learn to speak. These children should be taught sign language or an alternative computerized system.

Appropriate *eye and ear* screening should be done by the community doctor. Approximately 3% of children have a lazy eye which can lead to loss of vision in that eye if not corrected. These children display no warning signs even to the alert parents. The condition can be corrected, but for treatment to be successful, detection and treatment must be given around the age of 4-5years of age. Treatment usually involves wearing a patch over the good eye for periods up to 2 years to encourage the lazy eye to develop. Children do not like wearing a patch on the eye even intermittently, so a new approach is the use of glasses with an electronic shutter in the lens over the healthy eye. A tiny computer in a headband worn with the glasses, controls the shutter. The shutter closes over the healthy eye for short periods, forcing the lazy eye to function. Glasses should fit properly and not keep sliding down the nose.

Headache in a child, if persistent, should be fully investigated. The type, site and spread of pain, duration, frequency, intensity and factors relieving or exacerbating it must be evaluated. Whether or not a child is growing normally must be considered along with the other factors. Migraine is common in children and can be disabling. Many of the drugs used in adults are not licensed for use in children so it is important to use, at least initially, a basic pain-killer such as paracetamol.

The incidence of *hepatitis B infection* has risen in Ireland since 2000, probably because of the rise in sexual promiscuity and immigration from parts of the world where this infection is very common. Children must avoid early sexual experience. This can lead to sexual promiscuity. There may now be a need for the inclusion of hepatitis B vaccination in the childhood immunization programme and this now needs review.

Obstructive sleep apnoea may occur in children due to enlarged tonsils and can lead to disturbances in behaviour. If the child has a disturbed sleep pattern and does not seem rested after sleep do discuss this with your GP. Children with Down's syndrome are more prone to get sleep apnoea.

Be careful not to *over-treat* your children with medicine. Two of the main ingredients in over-the-counter (needing no prescription) cough medicines are possibly no more effective than taking sugary water, so a hot drink at night may be just as beneficial as the anti-cough medicine.

Premenstrual syndrome pain may be distressing in young women. This is probably due to wide changes in hormone levels with fluid retention. Usually there is no need for measures other than reassurance and salt restriction in the time leading up to the period. Some young women may need mild painkillers such as small amounts of paracetamol or anti-inflammatory preparations or on occasions may need tablets to inhibit ovulation such as the contraceptive pill.

10% of teenagers *sleepwalk*. Sleepwalking occurs in a non-dreaming sleep state. Sleepwalkers have unknowingly put themselves into situations of danger. People can do anything only without the 'fear factor', while sleepwalking. Your GP will advice regarding the necessary practical steps to take to combat this.

Approximately 5% of 3-4 year olds tend to *stutter*. Stuttering should be treated before the start of school, if possible. Your GP will advice regarding this.

Tuberculosis (TB) is still lingering in developed and underdeveloped countries. In cities like London, up to 50 people per week may develop the disease. In Ireland pockets of infection are still present. From time to time a patient with this condition is found, either diagnosed in school or by chance is detected by chest X-ray. Fortunately, a standard procedure can be quickly put in place to follow up potentially infected persons so minimal disruption to the school curriculum can be guaranteed. Sometimes people are resistant to medication and for these, long-term care is necessary and can be very discouraging. A form of TB resistant to drug therapy can occur with AIDS so it is important to avoid sexual promiscuity and casual sex. A new blood test to detect TB before symptoms appear may soon be available. Meanwhile vaccination against TB is recommended and very worthwhile.

Children should be *vaccinated* according to the recommended schedule. In the EU it is fortunate that the necessary vaccines of childhood are usually available in adequate supply, unlike the situation in parts of Africa. All vaccines are examined in clinical trials and only those with a positive benefit risk ratio are licensed. That does not mean that the vaccine will never cause side effects. No product is 100% safe for all people. In some individuals due to either genetic or environmental exposure conditions, the vaccine may cause side effects. Sometimes these can be life threatening, however the positive benefit risk ratio means that in a large population the benefits outweigh the risks of side effects. The measles, mumps and rubella vaccine (MMR) can cause side effects such as joint pain and reduction of blood platelets which are important in blood clotting. If there is a history of allergy or your child experiences any side effects from any vaccination tell your GP. While the MMR may also on rare occasions, cause encephalitis or inflammation of the brain, for the vast majority of individuals the benefit of vaccination outweighs the life-threatening risk of measles itself which can have devastating effects either in or out of an epidemic situation.

When booster vaccination is recommended against a particular bacterium it is usually a good idea to avail of this because sometimes immunity wanes following a change in vaccine supply or timing, leaving children vulnerable to infection.

Live vaccines should not be given to pregnant or immunocompromised individuals.

Each one of us has a unique individuality which should be nurtured. The way a country deals with 'special needs' individuals is a reflection of how it values all of its citizens. Students with special needs must be adequately educated. Almost 800 travellers are still living by the side of the road while almost twice this figure do not have permanent accommodation. How can travellers become well educated and move forward in the twenty-first century if their living conditions are so poor?

Specific accommodation programmes must be adopted for travellers as their present living conditions are definitely not acceptable however they must avail of opportunities to improve their status and avoid over-emphasis on old cultures. They must get education. All parents must be empowered to educate their children and all including the travellers must assume responsibility for this. Better understanding between travellers and settled people must be encouraged from childhood and both groups must be encouraged to respect the environment.

Key sentences: The teenager must find an identity in adolescence. Parents must be good role models. Parents must emphasize the dangers of alcohol and drug abuse. Parents must be tolerant and show flexibility but keep discipline.

12

In The Street and In Society

Although a lot of schools are now giving more attention to the environment, civic and social education is not assigned enough time in the school curriculum. These subjects should form part of the examination system. The streets of some of our cities are often littered with papers. Vomit from excess alcohol and urine can also be seen on occasions. Our cities badly need true group leaders. It will take a long time before Dublin becomes an 'A' capital but some good citizens can change almost any situation for the better. Improved civic awareness is needed in all social classes.

Some individuals will stay in dirty underwear for months with urine, faeces and semen all present. Keep yourself as clean as possible. To be clean is a wonderful experience. Dirt will lead to itch and to skin infection. The message to everyone must be to wash your hands with soap after going to the lavatory, before eating, after handling any dirty objects, chemicals or pesticides. Before dressing a wound, hands obviously must be washed. In Ireland 2006 cleaning facilities are available to all and basic clothes are very economically priced. Those sleeping rough should have access to washing facilities and clean clothes and they must be helped to rehabilitate by being housed and getting some form of employment. The will to rehabilitate and the belief that this can be achieved must be strongly encouraged.

In hospitals the methicillin- resistant staphylococcus aureus infection (MRSA) is present in ever-increasing amounts. Items in hospitals such as case notes, pens and computer keyboards act as reservoirs of infection. Hospital mattresses also harbour MRSA. Door handles and the toilet flush button are areas where bacteria can lodge. Once a bacterium sticks to an object it survives for many weeks. The infection can therefore be passed on indefinitely. MRSA is often transferred between patients due to poor hand-washing techniques by both staff and patients. It is essential for all to observe the hand-washing and other procedures laid down by the hospital in order to reduce infection. There is some evidence that silver can ward off MRSA. Silver-threaded machine-washable garments may soon become available in hospitals to counteract the MRSA. All visitors to hospital should observe hand-washing and other hygiene rules.

Body or breath smells are offensive. The smell of cigarettes can be nauseating. Excess alcohol can cause dehydration and make the breath very offensive. Smells of any kind should be avoided. The smell of poor hygiene, excessive perfume or aftershave are all situations to be avoided. Obviously not everyone appreciates the drenching smells of excess no matter how expensive the product. Gum disease causes bad breath and may be linked with heart disease, diabetes, smoking and osteoporosis. An offensive smell should be avoided by appropriate hygiene, dental care and avoiding smoking and excess alcohol.

There is growing fear that avian flu will soon affect humans. Avian or bird flu is a viral disease that causes illness in many species of birds. Avian flu has arisen from the appalling conditions in which birds are kept. While the condition has been highlighted in Asia, a lot of countries including EU members have been quite negligent in animal husbandry with some frightful conditions for poultry. If animals are treated poorly, kept in unnatural conditions or fed inappropriate food, sooner or later disease will occur. Most avian influenza viruses do not infect humans but the H5N1 bird flu can infect people in close proximity to the birds. It cannot currently be passed from human to human like influenza which affects people every winter. The big fear is that the H5N1 strain may mutate to a form that is easily transmissible to humans and between humans. Animal husbandry must be improved. Anyone travelling to infected countries should avoid going to farms or bird markets. It is always wise to avoid close proximity either in the home or elsewhere with anyone with a cough or bad cold.

Health of mind is as important as health of body. Positivity radiates from someone who feels at peace with himself and the world. There is a Russian proverb that says 'A kind word is like a spring day'. At work you may have to be tough in doing the 'right thing' but always be fair and be as kind as you can. Do not go along with the 'group' either at work or at play if you know that the group members are doing the wrong thing. Form your own opinion. Always listen to other points of view but make your own mind up about the correct way of doing things. Have respect for animals and for the environment.

Do not indulge in behaviour or gossip likely to cause mental or physical injury to people or animals. Always ask yourself "Would I like that to happen to me" ? Be careful when you get behind the wheel of a car. Speed can cause injuries and death. Abusive passengers are forcing bus drivers out of work every year. Spitting with all the risks of infection to others is not uncommon. Better education and knowledge of civic responsibility might in time change this mentality.

Fireworks can cause serious injuries to humans and animals. Guide dogs are often so traumatised by fireworks that they can no longer be used as guides. Their loss to a blind person is unimaginable. The sale of fireworks in shops or markets is illegal however the actual use of fireworks such as throwing a firework at a person, animal or property is not regulated. Fireworks are bought and used indiscriminately. Legislation may be needed to try to reduce serious unnecessary injuries to children and to animals. Take a lead and ensure that you do not damage a person, a pet or someone's property.

Remember that animals feel pain just like you do so try and be humane at all times. Ireland must improve its record with regard to the treatment of animals. Whether or not animal experiments should be conducted is a controversial question. Whatever the outcome we must all place great emphasis on the welfare of both farmed and domestic animals and in relation to the use of animals in scientific research. We all have a duty to adhere to the RSPCA principles of ensuring that animals are kept free from fear, distress, hunger, thirst, discomfort, pain, injury and disease with freedom to express normal behaviour. These principles must be communicated to children since children can be thoughtless and very cruel.

If possible do not smoke. Remember the halitosis (bad breath smell) and the smell from your clothes is offensive. If in spite of the bad smells you still must smoke do not drop cigarette butts on the ground. These are revolting! Stub out the cigarette and put into appropriate receptacle or litter bag.

Being too shy or too noisy can be bad for your health and well-being. Participate as fully as possible in society even if you have a tendency to be a loner! To participate fully in society you need to be able to read, write and manage your money. As many as 1 in 4 people in Ireland have difficulty with reading. Imagine how handicapped you might feel if you are unable to read or write. You hear about a suitable job but cannot write a letter of application. On the other hand, you can go anywhere and do anything if you have these basic skills. Parents must insist that their children get this basic education. Adequate resources must be provided for primary schools. It is the teacher's job to teach all children adequately and parents' responsibility to ensure that the children attend school. As Charles Dickens said in Nicholas Nickleby. "We hear sometimes of an action for damages against the medical practitioner who has deformed a broken limb in pretending to heal it. But what about the hundreds of thousands of minds that have been deformed forever by the incapable pettifoggers (Those who pay too much attention to unimportant details), who have pretended to form them"? A rather famous Irish-American actor now well past middle age has admitted that his education is deficient and wants to return to school to get more education. The message must be to avail of education no matter what your age. Learn to use basic everyday expressions and learn how to express yourself clearly with basic sentences. Attend free cultural experiences-art galleries, public lectures etc. Get a hobby, go on a course, make yourself more interesting whether this is by bird watching, hill walking, train spotting, picture painting or singing in a choral society!

Avoid being a workaholic. Work while at work. Get your work done. Take pride in it. If you have weaknesses such as poor spelling, correct these. If the work is boring resolve to get promotion or change jobs. Mix with co-workers but avoid familiarity. Do not gossip because someone will quote you and blame you for inventing stories. Once you have finished work, switch your mind to your hobby or to relaxation.

Avoid poorly ventilated atmospheres. Make sure that the hairdresser you visit uses clean towels and cleans combs between customers. If you like tattoos remember that these are a permanent fixture unless you can pay for laser therapy to remove them, so make sure you really want one and more importantly make sure that the establishment performing the procedure has clean sterile utensils. Tongue piercing is best avoided since the possibility of infection from the mouth bacteria or from non-sterile equipment, could be significant.

Key sentence: Improved civic awareness is needed in all social classes.

13

Cigarette Smoking

Smoking is bad for our health. Cigarettes contain tar, arsenic, cadmium and formaldehyde which are health hazards, and nicotine, which is addictive. As far back as 1938 it was reported that heavy smoking shortened life by at least ten years. Smokers have increased risk of cancer and the other big killers such as heart disease, lung disease and stroke. Mortality risks with smoking increase with the numbers of cigarettes smoked and decrease progressively with increasing number of years after stopping smoking. Even after one year the risk is very substantially reduced. Smoking cessation prolongs life.

Those who smoke at any time in their lives are five years older than their actual age. DNA (deoxyribose nucleic acid) carries the information needed for the maintenance of each cell of the human body. DNA sits on structures called chromosomes. Telomeres are tiny caps at the end of chromosomes which protect the DNA on the chromosomes from the ageing process. Telomeres shorten by a certain measure for every year smoked. In Ireland, although the percentage of those who smoke is down to 23.6% compared to 31.6 % in 1998 it is estimated that up to 20% of teenagers between 15 and 18 years, take up smoking. Rates for lung cancer in Irish women are double the EU average.

Smoking occurs more frequently in the less well off and the less-well educated. An Irish study has shown that mixed sex education increases the rate of smoking and drinking among teenage girls. Smoking can cause lung cancer, lung disease such as bronchitis and emphysema, heart disease, bowel disease and circulatory problems leading to stroke and amputations. Smoking can also increase resistance to insulin and may trigger diabetes. Emphysema is a condition where the lung air cells lose their elasticity and gradually the subject with this condition becomes unable to walk without extreme breathlessness. Lung cancer occurs when the genes controlling cell growth mutate and cells start to multiply. The mutation is due to smoking. While the effects of smoking on the lungs, the heart and the blood vessels have been highlighted on many occasions, it is also important to be aware of the damaging ageing effects of smoking on the skin. Smoking and passive smoking can also reduce fertility in men and women. Smoking reduces the success rate of fertility treatments. Smoking can decrease the blood flow to the placenta in a pregnant smoker. Male smokers have a higher risk of erectile dysfunction than non-smokers. Erectile dysfunction is an inability to achieve a satisfactory erection. Gum disease is higher in smokers.

Smoking can trigger asthma. Smokers with mild to moderate asthma are insensitive to inhaled steroids at low doses but may respond at higher doses, putting them at a further disadvantage since the use of steroids should be kept as low as is compatible with their beneficial effect. Steroids have great potential but should always be used in as low a dose as possible to prevent side effects due to osteoporosis, diabetes development and possible adrenal gland suppression. The adrenal gland is involved with supporting each one of us in times of stress so it is important not to suppress it. Smoking itself increase the risk of getting diabetes by making insulin less effective. Smoking affects the metabolism of drugs and vitamins and may cause decreased levels of vitamins in the body including decreased vitamin D, making the bones of smokers more susceptible to osteomalacia and osteoporosis.

Most people are aware of the hazards of smoking for the heart and the lungs, but until recently it was thought by some smokers and indeed by some researchers that the nicotine in cigarettes can help mental performance. A recent major two-year study showed that in fact smokers are 2.7 times more at risk of Alzheimer's disease than non-smokers. Alzheimer's disease causes loss of short and long-term memory and recognition. Presently there is no cure for Alzheimer's disease although drugs called cholinesterase inhibitors may be helpful in certain cases.

The big tragedy of smoking is that it frequently kills middle-aged people, knocking almost twenty-five years off their life span. A recent study has found that children who are exposed to environmental tobacco smoke may have a higher risk of developing lung cancer as adults. Parents must not expose their children to this risk.

Smokers must try to decrease the burden on hospital beds and avoid preventable disease by giving up smoking. A ban on smoking in the workplace in Ireland was introduced in March 2004. This was a courageous and landmark decision, not initially popular with everyone. In the past, unfortunate people who did not smoke, were obliged to earn a living in smoke-filled atmospheres and were afraid to speak out for fear of victimisation. A substantial majority of the workforce agree that the ban has benefited them and a large majority of people eating out in pubs and restaurants acknowledge that 'smoke-free' is better. The smoking ban will undoubtedly save many lives and reduce illness in the years ahead. Compliance with the ban is fairly high. It is noted however that at one of the airports, a cage-like structure, open to the elements has had to be erected as a smoking area for passengers waiting in its transfer terminal. It is hoped that other airports do not follow this example.

Nicotine can be very addictive and many smokers who try to quit suffer from strong withdrawal cravings that are based on a physical dependence. Some smokers attempting to stop, may benefit from nicotine patches that are used on the skin and release decreasing doses of nicotine, helping to ease the symptoms of withdrawal. Oral tablets are now also available to help the symptoms of withdrawal.

If you are not a smoker you must not begin to smoke. Be wise and avoid the nicotine, the halitosis (bad breath smell) and the bad clothes odour and keep the cigarette money for the new hobbies that you will commence in order to forget about smoking! If you are a smoker try to give up because of the health-damaging consequences for you yourself, the family, the home, the environment and the future generation. The adult smoker should be aware of the offensive smell that clings to their person, to their clothes and to their home, which no amount of air freshener can hide. Remember that the halitosis of a smoker can be particularly offensive and it is difficult to conceal. Never allow your child to smoke.

Key sentences: Smokers must try to decrease the burden on hospital beds and avoid preventable disease by giving up smoking. Remember that the halitosis (bad breath smell) of a smoker can be particularly offensive and it is difficult to conceal. Never allow your child to smoke.

14

Cancer

Most diseases result from a combination of both hereditary and environmental factors. The hereditary factors are called genes which are made of deoxyribonucleic acid (DNA). Each cell of the body contains thousands of pairs of genes. One gene comes from each parent. Genes are part of chromosomes. Nobody is perfect and almost everyone carries a potentially destructive gene. Cancer occurs when the genes controlling cell growth mutate and cells start to multiply. The mutations may be inherited or sporadic due to environmental factors such as smoking, hot food, obesity, alcohol or radon.

The gene for some types of breast cancers runs in families. 1 out of 500 women inherit the gene for familial breast cancer. Women with mutations of the BRCA1 and BRCA2 genes have a lifetime breast cancer risk of over 50%. Genes for certain bowel cancers and for a type of stomach cancer also occur in families. Approximately 1 in 200-400 people carry a gene that predisposes to a type of cancer of the bowel and some cases of ovarian cancer. In these familial cancers, disease tends to occur in young adults (less than 45 years and often less than 30 years). The thyroid gland is in the neck. A gene for a type of thyroid gland cancer can be detected in early life. In the US, children under 5 years with this gene, have their thyroid gland removed because of their susceptibility to developing cancer. Most breast and bowel cancers are however not known to be genetically inherited and non-hereditary cancer of the thyroid gland can occur following exposure to radiation such as occurred in the Chernobyl disaster. Many common cancers can be avoided if we choose our environment with care and avoid mutation-causing agents.

Exposure to bacteria and viruses early in life may have an important impact on health, affecting the later development of heart disease, diabetes, cancer and allergies. According to research, children who pick up infections from their peers early in life have the best defence against childhood leukaemia. This is because a strong immune system, developed in response to common infections experienced in childhood, can ward off leukaemia in those children who may be susceptible to this because of their genetic makeup. Cancer of the oesophagus or gullet is increasing in developed countries and although smoking and alcohol excess increase the risk of getting this cancer by almost 100%, there is also the possibility that during treatment of stomach ulcers, some native healthy gut bacteria which act as bowel protectors, may be eradicated, causing an increased risk of malignancy in the gullet. It is therefore important to try and avoid getting stomach ulcers or gullet problems by sensible food intake, stress reduction, moderate alcohol and not smoking.

Although genetics are important, most common diseases and cancers are not simply transmitted from parents to offspring. There is a continuous interaction between genetics and influences of the environment. Therefore disease manifestation usually requires environmental factors. Cancers of the lung, the breast and the bowel are common. It is thought that smoking may unleash bad free radicals which trigger inflammation and speed up the turnover of white blood cells. Smoking may also cause genetic mutations with blunting of the ends of chromosomes which are called telomeres. There will always be a few individuals who seem to escape the destructive potential of cigarettes. This might happen because smoking may cause lung cancer in one individual but not in another who may be less susceptible to the mutation-forming ability of the cigarette smoke. Cancer of the lung is higher in subjects, particularly smokers, in high radon areas. Consult a radon map from the Radiation Institute to see if your home is in such an area. If you do live in a high radon area ensure that a sample of house air is sent for analysis. A radon sump may be needed in the house.

Cancer of the breast is rising in most countries, mainly in females. The cause is not immediately apparent but the biggest risk factors include increasing age, having an early menstruation and or late menopause, not having children or having the first child after the age of 30 years. The contraceptive pill has not been proven to be linked with breast cancer but careful consideration should be given to the possible danger of any medication that is taken over a prolonged period of time in a healthy woman. The International Agency for Research on Cancer (IARC), a division of the World Health Organization (WHO), has indicated that the contraceptive pill may increase the risk of breast, liver and cervical cancer. Breast cancer may also be more common in women who are exposed to oestrogen such as hormone replacement therapy for long periods of time. A high saturated fat diet may cause breast cancer in one person but not another due to interaction of diet and genetic make-up. A high carbohydrate diet with lots of sugar may also be linked to a greater risk of breast cancer so a varied sensible diet is the wise option!

Routine mammography detects approximately 50% of breast tumors in women with the familial breast mutations BRCA1 and BRCA2 versus 75% in women without the mutation. Mammography is less successful at early detection in the familial cases because younger women where tumors are more difficult to detect, are involved. In the near future a more sensitive screening may be available to detect familial cases. Mammography screening for breast cancer is offered freely to certain age groups in certain parts of the country and should be availed of. This screening will be extended nationwide shortly. If there is a family history of breast cancer your GP will discuss suitable screening.

Bowel cancer rates are higher in Ireland than in the rest of Europe. This may be due to poor diet with up to recent times a relatively low consumption of fruit and vegetables, causing a lack of fibre. Fibre stimulates the bowel, making absorption of toxins less likely. If the bowel movement becomes irregular (continuous diarrhoea or constipation or any other abnormality particularly blood) for no apparent reason, discuss your symptoms with your doctor. He may suggest testing a sample of faeces for blood and or bowel imaging studies. If there is a family history of colon (large bowel) cancer or colorectal cancer ask for appropriate information regarding bowel examination. The rectum is the back passage. Examination of the bowel may reveal a condition called 'familial adenomatous polyps'. The polyp(s) can be removed and annual bowel examinations arranged.

All cancers appear to have an increased incidence in obese individuals. There are no miracle foods that prevent cancer but sensible eating and drinking, with regular exercise, can have a very positive effect on health. Once you have achieved a reasonably desirable weight for your height (See Table 1) then keep it there by avoiding binge eating and drinking, although full participation in the rare ceremonial occasion can be acceptable! It is prudent to eat plenty of fruit and vegetables, to drink adequate amounts of fluid and avoid constipation. Irritants in the diet include high fat (excessive saturated animal and hydrogenated margarine fats), and excesses of anything. It is wise to vary the diet while adhering to a sensible combination of fruit, vegetable, fat (small amounts of butter, vegetable or nut oil, fish and olive oil), protein (moderate portions of lean meat, fish and small chickens and turkeys) and carbohydrate (bread, potatoes, beans, pasta). Avoid nut oil if there is a history of nut allergy. Big turkeys and chickens should not be consumed as their fat content is often high because of their diet and absence of exercise, and their meat may contain residues of antibiotics. Fruit, vegetables and porridge supply fibre which may reduce the risk of cancer of the bowel. Pomegranate fruit (cheap and plentiful in autumn), broccoli, cabbage and cauliflower also have anti-cancer effects. By varying the diet no one constituent is eaten continually so for example traces of pesticide that can be found in some fruits, vegetables and meat are not eaten regularly. The body is a strong organ and can cope with traces of unwanted materials but not if these are allowed to accumulate.

Avoid irritants like smoking or the environment of smokers, or other pollutants. Cancer of the mouth and throat occur more often in smokers than in non-smokers and in those that drink alcohol in excess. Men who live in cities or towns and who smoke and drink are at most risk of developing cancer of the mouth and throat, however cancer of the mouth is increasing in women. In Ireland these cancers contribute to 1.5% (equivalent to 150 deaths) of all cancer deaths. This is unfortunate, because not only can these deaths be prevented but in addition, early treatment can be curative. Compared to other EU countries Ireland has a higher than expected cancer of the lip in males and a higher than expected cancer of the mouth in females. Cancer of the lip and mouth is high in the west of Ireland. This may be related to the fishing or farming industries. Binge drinking may be the cause of the sharp rise of mouth cancer especially in women. Oral sex may also be a factor. It is important for everyone to go immediately to your GP or dentist if anything unusual is noted on the lip or in the mouth.

Excess alcohol can cause oesophageal (gullet) cancer, laryngeal (throat) cancer and liver cancer. Liver cancer may occur in the presence of haemochromatosis a genetic condition where there is excessive iron absorption. There is a high incidence of haemochromatosis in Irish people. This affects the skin, the joints, the glandular system as well as the liver, and can cause difficulty with erections in males. It may cause diabetes. It can affect both sexes particularly males. If you develop a slate-grey or bronze-type skin pigmentation and or there is a family history of liver problems, it is wise to discuss a suitable blood test with your doctor.

Irish individuals expose themselves and their children to the risk of lethal skin cancer called malignant melanoma by being careless about their skin. Irish men working on building sites should ensure that adequate sunscreen and protective light clothing is used to avoid excessive and dangerous sun exposure. There is also some evidence that exposure to dioxins, which are produced by incinerators and by burning rubbish, can increase the risk of melanoma. Eye tumours can be caused by skin cancer and most of these could be avoided by using the appropriate sun-block for the skin type. Do not allow children to use sun-beds.

Cancer of the kidney is usually curable if detected early. Microscopic amounts of blood in the urine is often present so if you have an annual physical examination make sure you ask to have the urine tested for blood, sugar and protein.

It is desirable to prevent the onset of any cancer. However in those who have the disease the outlook and prospect of cure is improving all the time with new drugs. Breast cancer survival rates have improved enormously. The survival rates may be higher in some centres so the Health Service Executive (HSE) needs to ensure streamlined treatment protocols to ensure best care throughout the country. Certain breast cancers when examined at a detailed molecular level have receptor sites which respond to drugs which are specific for these receptors. Drugs which are called oestrogen inhibitors have already proved very useful in preventing breast cancer recurrence. Other drugs called aromatase inhibitors can help prevent recurrence of breast cancer in those subjects not responding to the oestrogen inhibitor. All licensed drugs have a positive benefit risk ratio meaning that benefits outweigh risks, however all drugs do not suit all people so your doctor will have to discuss the best one for you.

Treatment for leukaemias in both children and adults is very successful. Stem cell transplantation has also made possible the development of new therapy.

A biotechnology product grown from living cells has offered the prospect of a new lease of life to subjects with bowel cancer that has spread from its original site. Drug trials have shown a positive benefit risk ratio for this product. A new tablet which latches onto lung cancer and blocks a growth factor which encourages the rapid growth of the cancer, has now shown some good results in lung cancer patients. This may be beneficial especially where surgery is not possible.

Approximately one in fourteen men will get prostate cancer and this cancer has been linked to high cholesterol levels. More men die with prostate cancer rather than from it, however vigilance is needed in a patient with a newly diagnosed tumor. A high PSA (prostatic-specific antigen level) in the blood may be present and may have been detected at an annual physical examination. The prostate is examined by a rectal (back passage) examination. Depending on a man's age and on the microscopic appearance on tumor biopsy, it is recommended to have a PSA (prostatic-specific antigen level) blood test every 6-12months. If the PSA level is rising, or if the doctor on examination of the prostate gland feels any new areas of growth, then there is reason to suspect that the cancer is advancing and treatment may be indicated. There is now some evidence that the rate of rise of the PSA marker is the important parameter upon which to make a decision for further treatment. The blood test must always be taken before rectal examination as the examination itself may stimulate the gland and cause the PSA level to rise. More sensitive blood tests are being evaluated in the US. Radical treatment for prostate cancer can have fairly serious consequences such as urinary incontinence and possible impotence. Medical treatment which decreases male hormones which are called androgens may be useful although there are likely, as with all drugs to be some side effects. The good news is that in addition to new anti-androgen medical treatment, a new surgical procedure with much less prospect of side effects may soon become available. This combines high frequency ultrasound and laser ablation therapy.

Family history is important, however, it does not mean that for example because your mother died young from breast cancer that the same thing will happen to you! Preventive measures can be very effective. If there is a family history of cancer of any part of the body make this known to your doctor who will arrange suitable screening and follow-up.

There are higher rates of cancer referrals in lower income groups and it is still a fact that certain cancers occur more commonly in lower social classes with subjects less likely to survive than their counterparts in higher social classes. This is probably secondary to poor education, excessive smoking and poor eating habits. In women, cancer of the cervix (the neck of the womb) is known to be influenced by certain factors such as smoking and the number of sexual partners. Cervical smear testing (Pap testing) is used to detect abnormal cells in the cervix. In a recent survey in Dublin the number of women referred to a specialist for further investigation of abnormal cervical smears was higher at all ages in the lower income groups. Education about promiscuity and avoidance of smoking must surely play a role in decreasing this situation. A vaccine against the papilloma virus which causes cervical cancer is now available in the USA and may prove to be effective in decreasing cervical cancer.

The number of people who are free from cancer following treatment is higher than ever before and the number of cancer survivors have greatly increased in the last generation. Cancers in the mouth, throat, bowel, cervix and in the lung, are mostly preventable. The one big blot on the horizon is the increase in lung cancer deaths in women due to their taking up smoking. It is essential for all parents to encourage their children to avoid the lifestyle behaviours that cause cancer such as smoking, obesity, sexual promiscuity and excessive alcohol.

Key sentence: It is essential for all parents to encourage their children to avoid the lifestyle behaviours that cause cancer such as smoking, obesity, sexual promiscuity and excessive alcohol.

15

Alcohol

Many individuals who consume alcohol do so in moderation and light to moderate alcohol consumption may have a health benefit. The overall picture in 2006 is however one of excessive alcohol consumption in Ireland with a doubling of intake since 1970. While there are a variety of possible reasons for the escalation of alcohol intake, Ireland has always had a reputation for excess alcohol consumption. Reminders of this are everywhere, with Irish people often dying prematurely due to alcohol excess. In Ireland, alcohol seems to go 'to the head' in an extreme way, possibly because of our genetic makeup. Perhaps the Irish are suffering from 'genetic memory syndrome' following a traumatic event such as the famine. This can be handed down for several generations and result in modified gene expression. A propensity to alcohol abuse may have resulted from gene modification. Factors in the Irish such as brain chemistry, age when regular drinking began, beliefs about status achieved with drinking, party attendance, educational attainment, employment status, religious status, willingness of parents to supply money for alcohol at a young age, and lack of fulfillment either at work or at leisure may also be important. Unfortunately it was taught that Irish culture was inextricably linked with alcohol so children feel that alcohol excess is the 'norm' for our culture.

Alcohol misuse includes consumption of alcohol above the recommended daily, weekly or per-occasion amounts. The weekly number of units recommended is up to 21 for males and up to14 for females*. While there may be occasions when these are exceeded they should not be frequent as small amounts of alcohol are good for the health but excessive amounts are damaging not only to the liver and to the brain but can cause significant heart, blood pressure and gut problems and may trigger impotence.

*a measure equals a unit and is equivalent to half a pint of beer (about 270 ml), lager or cider or 1 small glass of sherry or of wine (150 ml) or 1 single tot of spirits (25 ml)

One bottle of wine is 7 units.

1 unit is equal to 15ml of pure alcohol or 12.8 gm alcohol.

Parents' attempts to allow children to drink in their company from a young age has been a misguided attempt to get over the strict taboo placed on alcohol consumption in the seventies, when in spite of the prohibition, underage drinking also occurred. Money was the limiting factor in the seventies. Now there is more money available and a greater choice of alcoholic drinks than in the past. Now because of excess there is a huge escalation in random violence in under-age drinkers because of the toxic effects of alcohol on the immature brain. In spite of this there are some parents, some vintners and some musicians who wish to give children greater access to pubs by opposing the liquor licensing laws that prohibit the presence of under-18s in bars after 9PM. The musicians point out that many groups playing in bars have members under 18 years of age. While the situation regarding the musicians may have to be given special consideration, it is appropriate that parents take responsibility for the welfare of their children. Late at night, children become restless and tired. Parents already merry and the worse for having imbibed too much alcohol may be unaware of their children's discomfort. Children assume that this is normal social behavior which in due course they will follow. This is not acceptable in a country where alcohol has caused many unhappy homes and premature deaths. Sleep patterns become disrupted. Attendance at work becomes disrupted. Alcohol-related problems cause family breakdown. Men are often disadvantaged by being seen as the main culprit in marriage breakdown and social or alcohol problems often results in them becoming homeless. All studies have indicated that dual parenting produces healthier, better educated children so every means possible to avoid social and family disruption must be advocated.

In the past when money was limited, alcohol excess was not that easy. Nowadays, with greater money availability, the impulse for socializing is greater than the work ethic. Alcohol consumption is far too high amongst young people where in many cases it is a cover-up for insecurity, loneliness and depression. Enjoyment for a lot of students is unfortunately linked to alcohol excess. It is somewhat dismaying that binge drinking is the 'norm' among university students with 3 out of 4 males and 3 out of 5 females involved in binge drinking. Third level education calls on each student's own resources to meet new challenges. The response through binge drinking indicates immaturity. It would also indicate that perhaps a lot of these students are insecure, lack self confidence and the coping skills for university and perhaps should seek alternative careers. The fact that there is so much money available to spend on alcohol is worrying. Student grants may not be deployed as wisely as they might be. It is also likely that students are working part-time to get money for alcohol. The end result is alcohol taken in excess, and stress near exam time. The focus on exams becomes lost since alcohol has clouded work, rest and play.

The subtlety of alcohol misuse is indeed quite frightening. At first alcohol may lift the spirits and the unknowing victim may feel that he is charming. The euphoria may lead to hospital admission, death, violence to others, or suicide. The phrase 'can't hold the drink' is somewhat inappropriate. Nobody can 'hold' excess alcohol without harming themselves or others, in one way or another. Random violence caused directly by alcohol excess is escalating. Binge drinking which is planned, coordinated and anticipated drinking is associated with all types of accidents and may lead to appallingly violent and terrifying behaviour and irresponsible sexual practices. A young man of 15 years was said to have acted totally out of character after drinking a large amount of vodka and subsequently raping a neighbour. Often, because of the effect of alcohol, women cannot remember whether or not sexual intercourse took place. The greater access to alcohol has lead to increased venereal disease and unplanned pregnancy. Irish women are making headlines as frequent binge drinkers and are now said to be committing more violent crimes because of this. Binge drinking has become so chronic in some areas that parish structures are disintegrating. One of our sporting organizations has warned that alcohol abuse poses the greatest threat to the success of Irish sports. This is indeed a serious situation and calls for urgent action.

Alcohol abuse occurs in all age groups or strata in society and this is relevant to our emigrant and indeed our immigrant population. The Irish in Britain are synonymous with alcohol excess even when they do not drink! A lot of the deaths, often prematurely, of the Irish in Britain are triggered by alcohol abuse. A coroner in the UK has called the English borough of Camden which has a large Irish community, the suicide capital of England. Irish-Americans have an alcoholism rate 2 or 3 times higher than the average. Many of our immigrants also seem to be having problems with excess alcohol.

Drink-drive deaths have increased. Every weekend there are usually at least three deaths from RTAs involving young men, and car crashes are one of the leading causes of deaths in adolescents. The contribution to these from excess alcohol intake is substantial. Figures for A and E departments indicate that many young drivers are admitted with injuries sustained while driving with blood alcohol levels of up to 300mg per 100ml. Alcohol impairs reaction time and other driving skills. The age at which alcohol-related deaths occur is getting lower with the death rate for young adults tripling since 1980. Drinking is now becoming widespread amongst teenagers with a median starting age of 13 years. Underage Irish girls have the highest binge-drinking rate in Europe and underage boys the fourth highest rate. The earlier a person drinks the more likely he is to become alcoholic. The typical male begins drinking heavily in his late teens or early twenties and has serious problems in his thirties. There is a close link between alcohol and depression and alcohol is a factor in approximately 65% of all suicides. Adults in the Republic drink almost twice as much alcohol as adults in Northern Ireland. Beer drinking has dropped by 15% in the last 10 years, with a large increase in wine consumption. Men make up 75 % of those treated for drug and alcohol abuse however with women now abusing themselves through binge drinking, the number of females seeking treatment for alcohol and drug abuse is set to rise.

Persons who misuse alcohol have elevated risks for a variety of health problems including violence-related trauma and injury. Contrary to popular belief, alcohol is not a stimulant but a depressant that slows down the central nervous system. It makes people less inhibited and able to carry out actions which they may later regret. Alcohol is known to affect the brain neurotransmitters in an area concerned with memory. It is not surprising therefore that alcohol may lead to memory loss. Over-consumption of alcohol leads to acute and chronic mental problems. Excessive alcohol is also a major contributor to illness and death from cancer, liver cirrhosis, bleeding from the gut, dilated heart and an increase in blood pressure leading to heart disease and stroke. In the presence of high blood pressure alcohol is best avoided. Alcohol excess can also lead to impotence.

Alcohol interacts with over 150 medications increasing the risk of driving and working while taking any such combination of drug and alcohol. The consumption of a combination 'lager with caffeine' designed to keep the consumer awake may promote the intake of more alcohol and is not advised. Alcohol consumed without food can cause a low blood sugar because alcohol inhibits the formation of sugar by the body which normally occurs when fasting. Food delays alcohol absorption and helps prevent a low blood sugar developing. A low blood sugar from alcohol intoxication could cause a fit or convulsion, in the past known as 'rum fits' from excess rum. The bad headache of a 'hangover' is due to dehydration of the covering around the brain and it is difficult to imagine why anyone would want this to happen particularly if it happens regularly. Alcohol is a metabolic poison as well as a depressant, which means it can affect normal body chemical reactions. The liver has to get rid of the alcohol and suffers particularly with excessive or binge drinking. Vitamin C can help the drinker to feel better. Grapefruit juice is helpful for the liver. After taking alcohol it is wise to take some still rather than fizzy water as the latter may increase alcohol absorption.

Data indicate that frequent drinking has harmful effects on the brain, and this may be more pronounced if people carry the gene called apolipoprotein- e 4 allele. Young males may perhaps be more vulnerable to the effects of alcohol than females because although the male brain may react slightly quicker than the female brain, the adolescent male brain matures less fast than in females, making males more likely to take risks. Autism, Fragile X syndrome and ADHD also occur more commonly in males, adding to their vulnerability at a young age. In some individuals, drinking excessively before the age of 50 may be linked to mental impairment later in life. All of these factors may now be contributing to the big increase in suicide. Alcohol has been found to be a factor in 60% of death inquests and causes more deaths than recreational drugs. Children should not be allowed to drink until at least 18 years of age. The adolescent brain is in many cases not fully mature until then and alcohol can harm the brain particularly the immature brain.

Some advertisements say that certain tonic waters can speed up the metabolism of alcohol, therefore it is implied that a high alcohol level may be brought under the legal limit. Such claims are dubious since it is very difficult to alter the metabolism of alcohol which is of the order of 10-15 ml per hour and hence the delay in recovering from acute intoxication.

Women because of their smaller size generally become intoxicated quicker and the alcohol tends to be more concentrated than in men. Binge drinking may thus be a factor in the sharp rise of mouth cancer especially in women. Young women must not allow themselves to become so drunk that there is a lack of insight and of inhibition resulting in danger to their long-term health and well-being.

Alcohol is known to cause chromosomal breaks in skin cells. It is not surprising therefore that it may cause abnormalities in the unborn foetus. The binge drinking culture amongst young women may be causing a rise in the number of babies born with mental disabilities. As many as one in 100 foetuses may be damaged by alcohol, causing learning difficulties in later life. Any female who becomes pregnant after consuming alcohol runs the risk of the baby being small for dates and possibly having teratogenic (deforming birth defects) effects from alcohol. Teratogenic effects include a small head, poor intelligence and epilepsy. Even more worrying is the fact that as many as nine babies in every thousand may be born with health problems due to alcohol, which can result in ADHD and poor coordination. Alcohol must not be consumed during pregnancy.

There are many people who feel that their lives are enhanced by alcohol. However for some, alcohol acts like a poison and must be avoided. In these people, alcohol causes problems and alcohol consumption leads to actions damaging to health and quality of life. For these individuals, 'one drink' will be harmful because many more drinks will follow, with all the inevitable consequences. These people are alcoholics. Twin studies have revealed that children of an alcoholic parent are more likely to become alcoholic themselves even if reared by an adoptive non-alcoholic parent. Genes and therefore heredity have a strong influence on alcoholism possibly by influencing tolerance to it. In mice a single gene controls the link between tolerance and alcohol consumption.

A few pints after work and a few laughs in the office may according to some economists be good for you. The key is however to keep social drinking at a moderate level and not to ruin the conviviality of the office by turning up late for work or not arriving at all the following day, due to a hangover. Sitting in the pub until closing time and drinking excessive alcohol is neither entertainment nor culture. If consumed, alcohol must be part of our diet and thus contributory to convivial social participation not 'our culture' as has been the mantra for many years. Alcohol problems can affect anyone. The WHO has developed the Alcohol Use Disorder Identification Test which can help a person identify if he has a problem with alcohol. The work supervisor must remain alert to changes in a worker's performance which may indicate a problem with abuse. That worker must be helped and rehabilitated. New legislation to be introduced in 2006 means some employees may face random tests for intoxicants.

The economic and social costs to the country of alcohol misuse are enormous. Studies have demonstrated that the incidence of alcohol-related problems is correlated to the amount of alcohol consumed and the greater the consumption, the greater the number of problems such as accidents, absenteeism and violence. A prevention programme is less costly than the treatment of dependent workers. Treatment for alcohol abuse needs to be community-based in order to facilitate early assessment and accessibility with prevention of a further downward spiral. For many people even a small intervention may prove life-saving. Treatment can take a variety of forms, with if necessary in-patient detoxification, counselling and the use of residential facilities. The public must be educated to understand the danger of excess alcohol for the drinker, the drinker's family and the public at large. A film highlighting the dangers of binge drinking and with a commentary and observations by young people will now be shown to second level students as part of the Social Personal Health Education subject taught at Junior Cert level.

Alcohol has taken its toll on many Irish sportspersons. It is quite amazing that alcohol is served throughout matches in the national sports stadium. The GAA's Task Force on alcohol and substance abuse has now been launched and banning of alcohol-related sports sponsorships must be recommended. Alcohol and sports do not mix. Alcoholism in adults is linked to youth drinking. In primary care, patients with past alcohol problems, young adults and high risk groups such as smokers and pregnant women may benefit from screening for alcohol misuse. Alcohol intake should be assessed and subjects advised on reducing alcohol consumption or if indicated, abstinence. Subjects should be assisted and motivated with the support needed for change. Repeated brief interventions can reduce problem drinking. Behavioural counselling could provide an effective primary care approach and future initiatives should focus on adoption of these practices into routine health care. Follow-up and repeated counselling, including appropriate referral if necessary to expert specialty treatment, should be given.

It will take many years before the habits of France, Spain and Italy of having a drink of wine with meals without further binging, are followed in Ireland. Avoid alcohol in the home unless this is well controlled. Be aware of your children's whereabouts and remember that under-age drinking tends to be ingrained from 15 to 16 years of age. There is little point in vigilance at home if children can get alcohol in a friend's house.

Parents must take responsibility for their children. Adolescents whose parents have problems related to alcohol or other drug use are three to four times as likely to develop such a problem themselves. The use of alcohol by parents is far more influential than giving lectures about its prudent consumption. Evidence from adoptive family and twin studies support a major genetic contribution to alcohol abuse with evidence that addictive factors for alcohol are transmitted in families. This does not mean that subjects with a particular genetic make-up will be alcoholics however that can indeed happen under certain influences such as alcohol excess or social rejection. In families with a history of alcoholism, prudence and avoidance of alcohol is wise.

Most EU countries have a legal limit for blood alcohol of 50mg per 100 ml. Ireland, Luxembourg, Malta and the UK have a 80mg limit while Sweden and Poland have limits of 20mg. With a 50mg limit, consumption of one glass (containing 150 ml) of wine or half a pint of beer (about 270 ml) would allow most people to stay below the limit. However even a very small amount of alcohol can impair the ability to drive safely so the wisest course of action in a country with such severe alcohol problems as Ireland, is to adhere to the slogan **'Never drink and drive'**. Random breath testing for alcohol and other drugs may soon be introduced in Ireland. The legal limit for breath alcohol is likely to be 35 microgram in 100ml of breath.

Addiction experts have plans to develop a patch that can control excessive alcohol consumption however this may be some way off. **Alcohol excess can change a decent citizen into a demented 'flasher'! Drink slowly so that your glass stays full longer, act sensibly and know when to stop.**

2005 was the William Rowan Hamilton year. WRH was born in Dublin. He was a great mathematician and a heavy drinker. Unfortunately not too many can combine greatness and excess alcohol and for a future generation moderation with alcohol intake must be a desirable aim. It is also important to understand that perhaps the Irish genetic make-up may not be compatible with alcohol, leading a substantial number to abuse it with devastating consequences to society. A certain 'coolness' and mysticism may have been attached in the past to alcohol excess, however in 2006 it is essential to remember that for full potential and productivity to be realized, a clear brain and a steady hand are necessary for all tasks. The dangers of 'drink and driving' but also the risks to health in general from alcohol excess and binge drinking need to be highlighted. Licensing laws need revision. Ongoing public education programmes based on the real dangers of alcohol must be maintained. It is ultimately however parental example which will change drinking habits in the young. Parents must take the lead and teach their children to be responsible regarding the use of alcohol.

Key sentences: For a future generation moderation with alcohol intake must be a desirable aim. Ongoing public education programmes based on the real dangers of alcohol must be maintained. It is ultimately parental example which will change drinking habits in the young.

16

Drug Abuse

The number of people being treated for drug abuse has risen dramatically outside the Dublin area. While heroin use fell in Dublin between 1998 and 2002 it increased outside Dublin. Some 25-45% of homeless people are thought to be dependent on drugs with alcohol still the primary drug of choice. A significant proportion of the homeless have both mental health and addiction problems. Evidence from adoptive family and twin studies support a major genetic contribution to drug use with some evidence that addictive factors for alcohol, cocaine, nicotine and cannabis are transmitted in families. While this does not mean that subjects with a particular genetic make-up will be drug users, that can indeed happen under certain influences such as alcohol excess or social rejection. In animals who are neglected early in life there is evidence of altered susceptible gene expression causing the animals to seek reward/ compensation through drugs. A similar occurrence in humans may or may not occur. Adolescents whose parents have problems related to alcohol or other drug use are three to four times as likely to develop such a problem themselves. Parents must look after their children. Drugs or alcohol alter the body and serious damage can be caused both in the short-term and many years later, if the subject survives. Almost one in five of all new cases treated for drug and or alcohol abuse are under 18 years of age. The brain has not even fully matured by 18 years of age so the potential for damage is great.

Cocaine use is thought to be one of the causes of the unexplained single-vehicle accidents involving young men drivers at weekends. Unfortunately a lot of these young men are ignorant about the hazards of cocaine and that of mixing drugs and alcohol. When people take illicit drugs they want the desired mental and emotional effects and ignore the damaging consequences that may result. Cocaine which is a stimulant drug can cause severe mood swings, increased heart rate and blood pressure and its use even on one occasion, can cause death. Even a short period of cocaine abuse can turn the most attractive face into a bloated, blotchy one that no amount of make-up can cover. More worrying however is the fact that cocaine causes heart and brain damage and can cause sudden death due to a heart attack. One person has died suddenly following a heart muscle disorder due to cocaine use. Brain scans have revealed that cocaine can damage blood vessels causing 'holes' in the brain leading to difficulty in thinking clearly with restricted blood flow precipitating seizures or stroke. Crack, the smokeable form of cocaine, is instantly addictive and can cause death through heart attack even after a single use. The smokeable form of the stimulant methamphetamine known as ice crystal meth. is a highly addictive substance being used in the US. It causes euphoria, hallucinations and leads to sleeplessness and psychosis. Psychosis is a severe mental disorder. Ice crystal meth. is particularly dangerous because it is made from chemicals rather than natural extracts. It is essential that this substance is not allowed into the country. Problems with drugs already here are so bad that a new more dangerous substance must not be tolerated. It is also essential that the so-called 'legal highs' available in the UK do not get distributed in Ireland. These contain a mixture of herbal extracts and synthetics and can cause significant mood alterations.

Teenagers begin with cannabis and volatile inhalants. 24% of 15-34 year olds have used cannabis (Also called grass, hashish, marijuana, pot) in their lifetime. Cannabis cigarettes can produce lung lesions which can lead to cancer. Cannabis even used occasionally can cause problems with memory and can affect coordination with resulting accidents. Smoking cannabis can give men breasts and decrease fertility. Chronic use of cannabis causes psychiatric/ schizophrenic-like symptoms while binge smoking of cannabis can lead to stroke. Inhalants are widely abused.

Some produce lung and brain damage which may be progressive. There may be loss of muscle control resulting in slurring of speech. Damage may also occur to the liver, heart and kidney. A few seconds of inhalation of air freshener has recently cost a 14 year old her life.

The use of opiates(heroin), 'ecstasy' (a hallucinogenic drug also called disco biscuits, rhubarb and custard) and amphetamines (a stimulant also called 'speed') tends to commence in late teens. Heroin can cause convulsions, coma or death. The pupil of the eye may become very small and the subject may appear lethargic and nauseous with frequent nodding. One dose of 'ecstasy' can kill or cause irreversible brain damage. A teenage girl recently died following two 'ecstasy ' tablets. She had not had these previously. Her companions did not suffer a similar reaction illustrating that illicit drugs can have lethal consequences which may not be expected. The wise course is always to remember that no two people are the same and never rely on the statement. "I had no side effects". Amphetamines have a high rate of psychological and physical dependence. They may cause agitation, hallucinations, convulsions, paralysis and possible death. Mental illness can develop which may not be reversible.

LSD or Lysergic acid diethylamide is a hallucinogenic drug, also known as 'acid' which can cause prolonged mental health problems. It can mimic the natural brain neurotransmitters and cause hallucinations such as seeing something that in fact is not there! Alcohol is known to affect the neurotransmitters so a combination of LSD and alcohol could be quite disturbing. LSD has led to suicide and accidents and can have very sinister effects in those who are mentally unstable.

Magic mushrooms include the liberty cap and can produce feelings of elation and euphoria as well as nausea and vomiting. Unfortunately in some subjects, particularly those with mental health problems, feelings of paranoia can be induced leading to psychosis. Liberty cap can be confused with more poisonous death-inducing mushrooms.

Although no social class is immune, the profile of drug users is that of poor education and unemployment. The highest rates of employment seem to be among those using ecstasy and cocaine. Those who use opiates and benzodiazepines (anti-anxiety drugs also called 'downers') have low rates of employment. Although benzodiazepines are in general safe drugs, addiction to them can cause problems.

Infected needles may transmit hepatitis B and C or HIV which causes AIDS. AIDS is not curable although drugs can keep it in remission. Other infections including fungal infections may attack the heart valve leading to long periods in hospital or to death.

Drugs taken by the pregnant woman can affect the newborn. Newborn babies may show withdrawal symptoms and behaviour symptoms. There is some evidence that a severe stomach abnormality in the newborn baby called gastroschisis follows the use of 'ecstasy' or cocaine by the mother in early pregnancy. Gastroschisis means that the baby is born with its abdominal wall open and all of the gut and internal organs are outside the body. No mother should risk this happening to her baby.

The difficulty of treating drug addiction has been highlighted by the US decision to establish 'Drug Courts' where drug addicts would be given the choice of rehabilitation or going to jail. The UK has also considered this regime and 'Drug Treatment Courts' are also been tried in Ireland. A pilot 'arrest referral ' scheme pioneered in the north inner city aims to turn young offenders away from a possible life of criminal behaviour. Treatment can take a variety of forms, with if necessary in-patient detoxification, counselling and the use of residential facilities. Unfortunately, once the brain circuits for addiction are established the motivational effects of drugs are as strong as the desire for food or sex. For the majority of drug abusers, who are often not in employment, a combination of treatment, support and education must attempt to halt further self-destruction. Research has indicated that people offered residential accommodation tend to do better than those who drift in and out of day care. Support programmes for children of drug users and one-parent families have been started. To prevent further drug addiction and alcoholism other causes of homelessness such as poverty, housing shortages, the high cost of rented accommodation, relationship breakdown or mental health problems all need to be addressed. People suffering with drug addiction must however want to kick the habit and not to continue to indulge it. Their responsibility is to avail of services to help them stop abusing themselves, their families and their surroundings.

Prevention is now more necessary than ever before since illicit drug availability is now increasing and at a lower cost than previously because of increased world-wide production. Therefore measures must be in place to tackle the supply and demand for illicit drugs. Prevention programmes in schools and in the workplace must remain the primary focus. The workplace mirrors to some extent the substance abuse problems of the community. New legislation to be introduced in 2006 means that some employees may face random testing for drugs and alcohol. Studies have found that people with substance abuse problems are more likely to abandon family and friends than to put their job at risk since the job supplies the money to pay for the drugs and or alcohol.

Parents need to be aware of the widespread availability of cannabis and cocaine and to emphasize to children the possible occurrence of grave long-term side effects following their use. The fact that premature death and disability are caused by the use of mood-altering drugs or alcohol abuse before the age of 50 years must be continually emphasised. Cocaine, 'ecstasy' and heroin must never be 'tried'. Amphetamines, cannabis and LSD can all lead to mental health problems and must always be avoided. Alcohol must be avoided completely in families with a history of alcoholism.

Some participants in competitive athletics may risk their health as pressure to win mounts. Some athletes may not be aware of the dangers of the inappropriate use of performance- enhancers such as erythropoietin, steroids, tetrahydrogestrinone, amphetamine and nandrolone. Lethal hormonal, heart, liver and kidney effects may be produced immediately or as a long-term consequence. Chronic intake may produce a considerably increased heart size and an increase in bad blood fats.

Workplace and school initiatives have the potential to reach the entire community and not just the working population. While all cases of illicit drug taking, alcoholism, suicide and sexual promiscuity will not be eliminated, education with primary prevention programmes in schools will at least give an insight into the perils of these activities and will lead to their reduction.

Key sentences: Once the brain circuits for addiction are established the motivational effects of drugs are as strong as the desire for food or sex. Therefore measures must be in place to tackle the supply and demand for illicit drugs. Prevention programmes in schools and in the workplace must remain the primary focus.

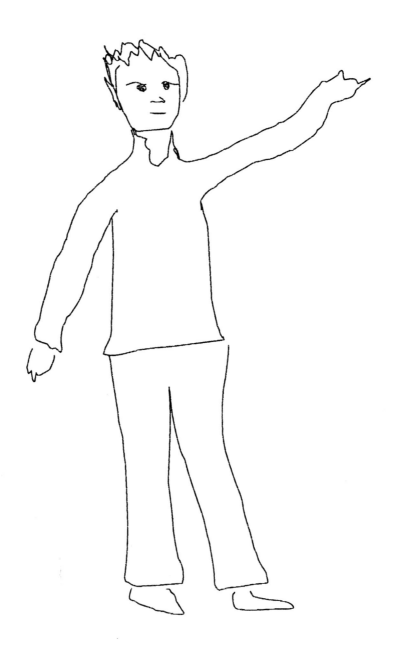

SAY "NO" TO DRUGS

17

Mother and Baby

The falling birthrate in Europe has galvanized governments into all sorts of schemes to encourage increasing family numbers. Women thus hold enormous power and influence and the saying 'The hand that rocks the cradle rules the world', is more appropriate than ever. This can certainly be said in Ireland where elections have been fought and won on the strength of women highlighting the need for childcare facilities! Ireland has one of the highest birthrates in Europe.

The conditions in the womb during conception and throughout pregnancy and breastfeeding have a profound effect not only on the baby at birth but also throughout its life. The mother and baby share the same blood supply so anything noxious to the mother will be even more noxious for the baby. All infections, food, drugs, alcohol consumed and cigarettes smoked by the mother may affect the baby. Thus complete dedication to the baby's well being demands a huge responsibility from the mother. The mother of course is usually totally dedicated to the well-being of the baby throughout the pregnancy and after pregnancy. She only wants what is best for the baby.

The GP and obstetrician provide extensive advice and support during and post-pregnancy and all pregnant women should discuss what they must do and also what they can and cannot do with regard to taking tablets, work, travel and leisure activity with their doctors.

The biologically optimal time for childbearing is said to be between 20 and 35 years.

Recently there has been an increase in babies born with a condition called gastroschisis, particularly to mothers under the age of 20 years. Gastroschisis means that the baby is born with its abdominal wall open and all of the gut and internal organs are outside the body. This condition may be due to drug abuse in the mother however the exact cause is not certain at this point in time. Avoid all drugs during pregnancy unless these have been prescribed for you by your doctor.

If there is a history of any disease in the family, any woman contemplating pregnancy should discuss this with her GP. Women with congenital heart disease must be sure to discuss this with their GPs since particular precautions may have to be taken during pregnancy. Women taking tablets for epilepsy must have these reviewed by their doctor prior to contemplating pregnancy. All pregnant diabetic patients need combined diabetologist /GP/ obstetrician care.

The well-being of mother and child is of paramount importance not only for their immediate health but also for their future health. It is mandatory therefore that there is adequate nutrition, absence of social problems including domestic violence, absence of any sexually transmitted disease and adequate advice for any physical or mental problems in the mother, before and during pregnancy. Pregnancy is not a time to experiment with diet. Stress to the unborn baby may result if undue emphasis is given to a particular nutrient. Stress in pregnancy must be avoided. Some recent research has shown that children born to stressed mothers may have elevated stress hormones for many years after they are born. Adequate rest is also important during pregnancy.

Folic acid (a B vitamin) supplements should be given as early as possible in the pregnancy to prevent neurological problems, called neural tube defects, in the baby. Widespread education about the benefits of taking folic acid during pregnancy has not increased consumption amongst Irish women who carry a high genetic tendency for neural tube defects. Neural tube defects occur in 27/10,000 Irish children compared to 16/10,000 European children. Even women who have relatives who gave birth to affected children do not take the necessary folic acid supplement. In fact almost 70% of first-time mothers do not take folic acid prior to conception despite its proven ability to halve the incidence of neural tube defects. The reason for this apparent forgetfulness is that the woman often does not realise that she is pregnant until a pre-natal visit is arranged. The sensible approach should be that any woman who suspects that she is pregnant, particularly if there is a family history of spina bifida or related disorder, should immediately take a daily 0.4mg dose of folic acid. *This dose of folic acid is safe however excess of any vitamin supplement should never be taken as excess may do more harm than good.* While the Food Safety Authority has recommended adding folic acid to flour this proposal has not yet been accepted.

Particular attention must be paid to the mother's *pre-pregnancy vaccination* schedule. Pregnant women are tested for their immunity to rubella (German measles). If a non-immune pregnant woman gets infected with rubella the baby may be born with heart defects, deafness or cataracts so it is important that this situation is avoided by appropriate childhood or adolescent vaccination. Vaccination against rubella must not be given during pregnancy.

Appropriate history, examination and blood testing should be undertaken in all pregnant women to avoid the transmission of infection to the foetus (unborn baby) or newborn baby. All pregnant women are screened for syphilitic infection. Syphilis is an infection acquired by sexual intercourse. It increases the risk of HIV infection by making it easier for the HIV virus to get across damaged membranes. All pregnant women must be tested for HIV infection. All pregnant women should also be tested for hepatitis B as a considerable proportion of children infected with hepatitis B, become infected from their mothers. If the mother is positive for any or all of these infections appropriate treatment of the mother is required. The newborn infant will also require treatment for HIV infection and hepatitis B vaccination.

Pregnant women who never had *chickenpox (varicella)* should avoid exposure to patients with chickenpox or shingles. Shingles, also called herpes zoster is caused by the same virus as chickenpox. Pregnant women who have had chickenpox in the past are immune to the infection. Their antibodies will also protect the baby. Mothers who are not immune and who develop chickenpox during the first 28 weeks of pregnancy may become very unwell with pneumonia and may infect the foetus. Chickenpox rash is often the first sign of illness. The rash occurs most commonly on the face, scalp and chest and sometimes in the mouth. Spots which are dark red pimples, appear over a 3-day period. Blisters develop on the pimples after a few hours. Prompt treatment of the mother with antibodies to the virus and an antiviral drug is required. Maternal varicella in late pregnancy can cause infection of the newborn baby. Protection of the newborn baby by treatment with antibodies to the virus and an antiviral drug is required.

Primary *herpes infection of the genitalia* (herpes genitalis) in early pregnancy may rarely cause foetal abnormalities. Primary means that it is the subject's first experience of herpes simplex infection and therefore she has no immunity. This usually occurs through sexual contact including oral sex. There is no cure for genital herpes although antiviral ointments can reduce the skin sensitivity and pain experienced and recurrent attacks tend to become less painful. A herpes rash present in the mother when the baby is due to be born can cause the baby to be infected, therefore a Caesarean section would need to be performed to avoid neonatal herpes. Neonatal herpes though rare is a very serious infection.

Listeriosis is a rare infection which is thought to be due in many cases to eating contaminated food. In healthy people the infection resembles a mild influenza. In pregnant women, it may affect the foetus and can lead to miscarriage, still birth or severe illness in the newborn infant. Pregnant women should avoid foods that can become infected such as pâté, brie, camembert, blue vein type cheese and ready-to-eat poultry unless this is thoroughly reheated.

Smoking can affect the blood supply to the foetus. A pregnant woman who smokes may damage the arteries of the foetus. The blood vessels from foetuses who died pre-birth, and from cot-death infants often show evidence of furring of the arteries. There is also evidence that smoking during pregnancy can damage a baby's lung and children of mothers who smoke have smaller airways with a 20% lower airflow than children of non-smokers. Smoking can result in low birth-weight babies and smoking causes an increased risk of miscarriage, stillbirth and cot death.

Pregnant women who drink *alcohol* can cause damage to the foetus thus placing a future generation at a disadvantage pre- birth. Many women unaware of their pregnancy continue to drink alcohol during the initial weeks of pregnancy. In Ireland up to 78% of pregnant women admit to drinking alcohol during pregnancy. The amount consumed can vary up to 6 units per week*. More than 300 babies are born each year in Ireland with Foetal Alcohol Syndrome and this figure increases to more than 1700 if all alcohol-related neurological disorders are included. This condition may present as birth malformations, lack of growth, or as a hyperactivity disorder. Research has shown that even one drink a week in pregnancy can trigger behavioural problems in children. As safe levels of alcohol during pregnancy are unknown pregnant women should not drink any alcohol. All pregnant women and women contemplating pregnancy should be informed of the harmful effects of alcohol on the foetus.

*a unit is equivalent to half a pint of beer (about 270 ml), lager or cider or 1 small glass of sherry or of wine (150 ml) or 1 single tot of spirits (25 ml)

One bottle of wine is 7 units

1 unit is equal to 15ml of pure alcohol or 12.8 gm alcohol.

During pregnancy, the mother gains between 25 and 35 pounds on average, mostly in the third trimester. Obese women should gain less and underweight women should gain more. A well-balanced diet is necessary in pregnancy as for non-pregnant individuals. A small amount of chocolate may be beneficial to mother and baby but small means small (one or two squares of chocolate on alternate days) and nobody must eat because "I felt low in sugar"! The higher the cocoa content in chocolate the better it is! Chocolate contains vitamins and minerals and can be quite calming or even act as an antidepressant! The cocoa content may be a useful ant-oxidant preventing dangerous free radicals forming in the body.

Women contemplating pregnancy should avoid *obesity* as obesity in the mother is linked with a greater risk of diabetes during pregnancy and a big baby. Ideal baby weight is between 6.5 and 8.8 pounds. Babies who have a high birth weight (greater than 9 pounds or 4.1 kg) have a higher risk of obesity later in life and infants who are underweight at birth (less than 6.2 pounds or 2.8 kg) but who catch up rapidly could also be more likely to grow into obese adults. The small baby has learnt to use its food supply with great efficiency. Consequently when after birth the baby receives a plentiful supply of food it tends to lay down fat stores which in time contribute to obesity. Obesity can lead to diabetes.

Research has shown that eating oily fish once a week during pregnancy may protect the baby against asthma. Eating fish is also beneficial to mother and child as it has fatty acids (Omega −3) which are essential to the body and to the development of the baby's brain and eyes.

Liver is not advised during pregnancy because it contains too much vitamin A which may be harmful for the foetus. Vitamin E supplements should not be taken during pregnancy.

Tablets other than the mineral or vitamin supplements advised by the GP should not be taken during pregnancy unless these have been prescribed for a medical condition such as high blood pressure. Herbal remedies or homeopathic medication should not be taken.

Pregnancy is a normal event and generally most employments cause no increased hazard to mother or foetus. Night shift work is probably best avoided during pregnancy. Advice should be sought if there is significant exposure to X-rays, gases, drugs or insecticides. Pregnant women should obviously avoid heavy lifting and exposure to vibration. Pregnant women in jobs with no toxic risk usually can continue working for as long as they wish however if any complications arise, permission to leave work early, must be given. In pregnancy all the usual exercises can usually be followed such as walking, dancing and swimming or cycling if practical. Forbidden are skiing, mountaineering or water-skiing.

Women with diabetes can have a normal pregnancy and a healthy baby provided their blood sugar is kept well-controlled by diet and insulin. Mothers are usually very dedicated to this and maintain very tight control in order to protect their unborn baby.

Ireland's breastfeeding rate of 1 in 4 women is the lowest in Europe. Babies who are breastfed have a significantly lower risk of death in the first year compared with non-breastfed babies. Breastfed babies have also been shown to have lower rates of infection. Breast feeding is said to decrease the risk of the baby developing intolerance to gluten a protein which is found in wheat, rye, barley and oats. Coeliac disease is a disorder of the small bowel caused by gluten intolerance. Babies should be breast-fed if possible but no mother should be made feel guilty if this is not possible. Breast milk contains a good source of iron. Cows' milk can be introduced at one year.

The Department of Health must continue to emphasize the risks of not breastfeeding. Breast feeding continued for one year is the best way to feed the infant however infant formulae are safe alternatives. It is essential that the formulae are reconstituted properly per directions since infants can dehydrate quite quickly with over-concentrated feeds. If soya milk is used ensure that it is an infant formula. Infant formulae are fortified with iron. Solid food is usually introduced between 3 and 6 months.

Vitamin D deficiency can occur in breast-fed babies. A big proportion of vitamin D is formed in the skin and during the winter months the mother may not receive adequate skin supply. It is sometimes necessary to give vitamin D supplements to the mother during pregnancy and breast-feeding if the dietary supply of vitamin D from eggs and fish is low. It may also be necessary to supplement the diet of a child up to the age of 5 years, with vitamin D. The GP will advise regarding the need for supplements.

Babies born by Caesarean section may have a greater risk of developing infection and allergy to cow's milk, eggs, fish and nuts, possibly because these babies do not have the experience of the normal bacterial flora in the birth canal. They also may be more at risk of tooth decay due to a cavity-causing bacterium. The demand for Caesarean sections seems to have increased in recent years and now accounts for one in five births in the UK.

500 pre-term babies are born in Ireland each year. The mother may notice that the baby tends to avert its gaze to protect itself against excess stimulation. These babies need to gain about 0.15kg per week in weight in order to thrive. A lot of GP support is necessary.

All new mothers should be made aware of the dangers of cot death (SIDS or sudden infant death syndrome)and the danger of sharing a bed. Infants should be put to sleep on their backs only, not on their sides. The safest place for the newborn baby to sleep is in the mother's room in a cot. Sharing a bed with parents is forbidden and it is obvious that no smoking should occur at any time. Soothers or pacifiers (or dummies in the USA) can also reduce cot deaths according to the American Academy of Paediatrics however these may also cause the baby to be less interested in breast feeding so they should not be used excessively. Recently concern has been expressed by mothers that putting the baby on his back may cause him to develop a flat head. In fact some mothers assumed that the baby should be on his back all of the time! This is of course false and the baby should assume any enjoyable position when awake. Lying on his back is the mandatory position only for sleeping. If while awake, the baby does come into the mother's bed it is important to ensure that the baby cannot get caught between the mattress and the headboard as small babies can get into awkward positions and get injured.

Children should be vaccinated. During a measles outbreak MMR may be given to children as young as 6 months of age. Children vaccinated before their first birthday should receive MMR at 15 months.

Tuberculosis (TB) is still lingering in developed and underdeveloped countries. Vaccination against TB, often at birth is still highly recommended as pockets of infection still occur.

The incidence of hepatitis B infection has risen in Ireland since 2000, probably because of the rise in sexual promiscuity and immigration from parts of the world where this infection is very common. The need for the inclusion of hepatitis B vaccination in the childhood immunization programme may need review.

A mother's intuition is said to be more important for her child's future than social status or wealth, with children whose mothers could read their feelings scoring higher in language and play tests. A study has indicated that if a mother understands her baby at 8 months it bodes well for the child's development by age 2 years. Baby milestones should be known to all mothers.

Early diagnosis of deafness is vital. Up to three months there should be a little jerk of the body or blinking in the presence of loud sounds. Between 3 and 8 months there is recognition of familiar sounds especially the mother's voice. Between 9 and 14 months baby listens to sound attentively. Between 14 and 24 months there is a quick response to faint sounds and these are localized. At 24 months speech is present. Boys are slower to talk than girls.

If a mother suspects that her child has problems with vision or eye movement, special hospital equipment can detect this.

The mother must ensure that a range of good quality sensible foods are taken by herself and the toddler (1-3 years of age). A routine of three meals a day should be introduced. One cup of juice and about three cups of milk are adequate per day. Soft drinks can be taken occasionally. Avoid lollipops as these have too much sugar and crisps as these have too much fat and salt. Snacks such as cheese, fresh fruit, yoghurt, meat sandwich and water are better. Cows' milk can be introduced at one year. Introduction of cow's milk in the first twelve months and excessive cow's milk during the first three years may lead to poor intake of other food and to iron–deficiency anaemia.

The average weight gain in the first year of life is about 6.5 kg. This decreases to approximately 2.5 kg per year in the second and third years.

In pregnancy some women may have loss of scalp hair. The latter usually recovers after pregnancy.

Post-natal depression may affect one in ten women. It can last from a few days to several months and can be mild or severely incapacitating. The more severe form occurs in approximately 1 in 1000 women. Symptoms may include constant tiredness, sleeping problems, tearfulness, lack of interest in the baby and panic attacks or other irrational thoughts. Any woman with these symptoms should see her GP.

Key sentences: The well-being of mother and child is of paramount importance not only for their immediate health but for their future health. As safe levels of alcohol during pregnancy are unknown pregnant women should not drink any alcohol.

18

Sexual Disease

 $\mathbf{V}$ enereal disease which is disease communicated by sexual intercourse, is increasing significantly in Ireland. HIV and AIDS the disease caused by HIV infection can be communicated by sexual intercourse or by blood and is an ever present threat for both homosexual and heterosexual people. It is estimated that one third of those with HIV are unaware of their infection. HIV-positive women can transmit the virus to the unborn child. AIDS is not curable but can be held in remission with a combination of drugs.

A recent survey has found that 25% of Irish adults think it is acceptable to have more than one sexual partner. Sexually-transmitted infections are increasing in the over-50 year olds who are often totally unaware of the cause of their symptoms. Binge drinking may contribute to poor judgement, to 'one-night stands' and to venereal disease. It is also important for anyone travelling abroad to be aware that 'one-night stands' can lead to any type of venereal infection since AIDS, hepatitis B and C and syphilis are now extremely common in some countries. If following sexual intercourse you have sores or a rash, an unusual discharge, pain during sexual intercourse or on passing urine, you may have a venereal infection.

For the past few years syphilis has reappeared. Syphilis is a venereal disease which if untreated may appear in almost any organ of the body many years after the initial infection. While syphilis is still fully sensitive to the antibiotic penicillin, a new mutant, antibiotic-resistant strain is common in patients attending Dublin clinics. This will have implications for treatment of sexually-transmitted disease, needing a combination of drugs rather than a single drug to treat both the relatively common chlamydia infection and syphilis. Chlamydia is a venereal disease affecting men and women, often with no symptoms, which can lead to infertility, particularly in women. Testing for chlamydia is straightforward with PCR urine testing being as informative as samples obtained directly from the cervix. A nasal vaccine for chlamydia may soon be available. Persons engaged in high-risk sexual behaviour may have helped the spread of the mutant strain of syphilis.

AIDS weakens the immune system and allows diverse infections including a rather resistant form of tuberculosis to attack the body, particularly the lungs, the brain, the blood and the eye. While there are now new drugs available to treat AIDS, these drugs are not curative and at best allow the patient a long remission from symptoms. The drugs usually have to be taken as a combination to avoid the development of resistance. The good news regarding AIDS is that the HIV may be weakening and recent work has shown that stored samples of the most dangerous strain from the 1980s were more infectious than samples from 2002.

Sexual behaviour can lead to cancer of the cervix, HIV infection, AIDS, hepatitis, infertility and abortion. It has a huge effect on premature death in the young and may cause prolonged disability. The US by contrast with Ireland and the UK has for the past few years become more conservative sexually with substantially decreased tolerance of sexual promiscuity. Counselling for teenagers has taken the attitude that there is little point in telling young people not to have sex if in a sentence later one adds " If you must have sex this is how to go about it". Teenagers in the US now seem to accept that sexual activity is really an adult activity and they want to remain free of sexually-transmitted disease for as long as possible.

Genital herpes most often arises from sexual contact including oral sex. In the male the penis is the most frequent site of infection. In women lesions may occur on the vagina or in the cervix. In both sexes, lesions may spread to surrounding skin sites. Unfortunately, genital herpes can cause recurring episodes of itching or painful genitals and there is some risk in pregnant women of premature birth or miscarriage. Women with genital herpes infection can transmit the disease to their partner even when they themselves have no obvious lesions. However, although these women have no obvious genital lesions they may have other symptoms such as pain or discomfort on passing urine, a vaginal discharge or swelling of lymph nodes in the groin area. Although no treatment can cure herpes, early diagnosis of herpes infection is essential. It is important to get antiviral treatment which can relieve the painful lesions and to get advice to avoid passing on the infection. Herpetic lesions on the genital area can increase the risk of transmission of HIV infection. Pregnant women who suspect that they may be infected should see their doctor for assessment.

A considerable proportion of sexually-active young adults are unaware of the infectiousness of ano-genital warts caused by a papilloma virus. They are also unaware that certain types of papilloma virus may cause cancer of the cervix later in life. In many countries sex education with portrayal of 'protected' sexual intercourse as an ordinary non-special experience has been found to actually encourage sexual intercourse and sexual promiscuity amongst teenagers. Children exposed to sex on TV are more likely to try and experiment sexually themselves so parental guidance must be fair but firm. Parents must ensure that their children do not commence sexual activity too early. Early sexual intercourse increases the risk of cervical carcinoma and may cause many emotional problems.

Gonorrhoea, a venereal infection which can lead to infertility in females is also increasing rapidly. Hepatitis B and C are infections transmitted through contaminated blood or by sexual intercourse. Both can lead to lifelong illness and premature death from hepatitis and liver cancer.

In the near future a vaccine against the papilloma virus which causes cancer of the cervix, may become available in Europe. Even when this vaccine becomes available it will still be necessary for all sexually active women to have some form of cervical screening. Currently, although some areas of the country are carrying out cervical screening programmes, there is no national scheme in operation. The traditional screening test is called a Pap test which is done by the GP, in women's clinics and in hospitals. This can successfully detect abnormal cells that lead to cervical cancer. Combining the Pap with a test for human papilloma virus provides a more accurate screening tool for cervical cancer. Screening is important, bearing in mind that in Ireland today there is a high incidence of sexually-transmitted disease and a lower age at commencement of sexual intercourse, both being contributory factors in cervical cancer. Many women however find the Pap procedure uncomfortable and some even avoid the test. Recent research has indicated that women may soon be able to carry out an alternative test at home. This is presently undergoing study trials. It works by microchip technology to measure the electrical resistance in tissues which is altered in the presence of abnormal cervical cells. The microchip is the size of a tampon and can be inserted by the woman herself into the vagina for 10 seconds in order to get a reading. The chip is then sent off for analysis. If trials are successful the microchip may become available as an alternative to the Pap test.

Key sentences: Sexual behaviour can lead to cancer of the cervix, HIV infection, AIDS, hepatitis, infertility and abortion. It has a huge effect on premature death in the young and may cause prolonged disability.

19

Obesity

Serious fatness or obesity is present if the waist size is greater than 35 inches (approximately 88 cm) in women and 40 inches (102 cm) in men. This is equivalent to having a body mass index (BMI) ≥ 30. At least 15% of Irish people are seriously overweight with BMI greater than 30. A much larger number of people have BMI in excess of the recommended 19-25 range. While the main goal of the HSE must be to reduce the number of subjects with waist size of 35 inches plus, primary care must strive to prevent those in the 25-29 range from getting bigger. Exercise must play a major role.

The phrase' It's a funny old world' is often used and can be appreciated quite well in the case of obesity. While half the world is starving, another half is striving either to eat as much low calorie food as possible without gaining weight or to get an operation to remove weight. In parts of the underdeveloped world and in the midst of famine, women are actually force-fed until crippled with obesity because custom says that they are more desirable sexually that way. In children, obesity carries with it increased risk of high blood pressure, diabetes and low self-esteem. Obesity is the big disease of the twenty-first century. School uniforms have increased substantially in size in the UK, and in Ireland, advertisements like 'Extra-large Communion frocks' available, can be seen in shops. Obesity, diabetes and heart disease are all interlinked. A US study has shown strong connections between eating 'fast food' two or three times per week and resistance to the action of insulin, with resulting weight gain and risk of diabetes and heart disease. A considerable number of patients with heart disease have abnormal sugar regulation. Obesity is overtaking smoking as the leading cause of preventable disease.

Being overweight is due to eating more food than one can use, without working off the calorie excess through exercise. There are genetically determined syndromes in humans which are associated with obesity such as the Prader-Willi syndrome but these syndromes are rare and human obesity is not due to a genetically abnormally low energy expenditure but by eating too much food and not taking adequate exercise. Unfortunately as the waist increases so does the risk to health. Fat on the abdomen or belly is more dangerous for your health than fat on the buttocks. Eating too much for one's calorie expenditure on a daily basis, can lead to a gradual weight gain.*

*More than 5 kg in 5 years

1 kg = 2.2 pounds

Lack of exercise increases the risk of obesity. There is a greater risk of obesity in the less well-off and the less well-educated. Women tend to become obese more frequently than men and women who have had several children tend to be fatter than women with less children. However, women with several children who have high educational level tend not to become obese possibly by increasing their exercise in order to counteract excess calorie consumption. High alcohol intake with an unhealthy lifestyle contributes to obesity with 'beer belly' causing excess fat to accumulate in the abdomen. Obese young women age faster than their non-obese contemporaries. Telomeres, which protect our genes by sitting on the end of the chromosomes, get damaged faster in obesity because the excess fat unleashes free radicals causing inflammation.

Smokers tend to gain some weight on stopping smoking for a variety of reasons including the fact that after stopping smoking the taste buds operate better and extra food is consumed. The benefit of giving up smoking is far greater than the risk of gaining weight and sensible eating with exercise can avoid any significant increase in waist size. Obesity increases with age because of decreased activity, however young children are now becoming obese due to excessive snacking in front of the TV. Lack of sleep may also cause people to overeat.

Being obese increases your risk of experiencing a variety of serious health problems and the possibility of premature death. Obesity causes people to get disease of the heart, gut, brain (strokes) and breast more frequently and earlier than non-obese individuals. Obesity frequently leads to high blood pressure and in many instances, particularly where there is a family history of the condition, to diabetes with all its health risks. Excessive fat deposition may stress the gall bladder and will cause damage to joints with resulting poor mobility. Obese subjects often need hip replacements and are at increased risk of certain cancers. Obesity causes a fatty liver. Obese women are more likely to have problems in pregnancy and to suffer with depression and attempted suicide. Obese subjects may suffer with obstructed nasal breathing and tend to snore heavily, with some likelihood of impairment of brain circulation. It is therefore possible that obesity in middle age increases the risk of dementia later in life. Fat people have difficulties with clothes, walking and seating on public transport.

People who overeat to extremes do have at the very least, a psychological problem and need help to overcome this addiction. However, in a world where a huge population is overeating because of food access and excess and an even larger population is dying from famine the morality of surgery for obesity may be questioned. Sensible eating, avoidance of everyday dietary excess, and exercise are the best methods of keeping reasonably fit and avoiding fat accumulation. Gradual loss of weight is ideal since rapid weight loss may cause worsening of 'fatty' liver disease. Some 'slimming' tablets may be helpful and have a role to play.

Surgery may be useful in selected morbidly obese patients (BMI more than 40). This requires interaction between patient, surgeon, physician and dietician. Gastric bypass involves making a pouch of small volume by stapling across the stomach and connecting the lower part of the small bowel to this, bypassing the main stomach and the upper small bowel. Bypass can cause about 60% of excess weight to be lost by about 18 months however there is a substantial risk of nutritional deficiencies arising because of malabsorption and this must be taken care of by appropriate supplementation. Gastric banding is another form of surgery where a small stomach pouch is formed by a Dacron type band. With gastric banding 36kg may be lost over one year and while nutritional deficiencies may occur these tend not to be as great as with bypass. After surgery, subjects must adapt to dietary restrictions. Usually they can manage to do this and a substantial number do not regain weight.

Surgery may be life-saving particularly in subjects so obese that the risk of breathing problems such as obstructive sleep apnoea syndrome is high. In such patients surgery improves not only the breathing problem but also improves diabetes, blood pressure and fat disorders so essentially it reduces the risk of heart disease and heart failure. While surgery can have a satisfactory outcome in certain patients, it is important to remember that the morbidity immediately after surgery is high and can be nearly 10% owing to possible surgical or medical complications. The aim must be to prevent an individual becoming so fat that surgery is necessary. *Once compulsive eating is noticed by a relative or partner, counselling, psychological and psychiatric help should be obtained.*

The aim for all of us must be to create awareness of the seriousness of being obese and to empower all to do something about it. Access to food mountains does not mean eating a mountain! Obesity can be reduced by exercise and sensible eating. If possible leave the car at home and use public transport. One must not be obsessed by trying to achieve an ideal body weight. Rather achieve a stable weight than a fluctuating or steadily increasing weight. Eat moderate amounts of good quality basic food rather than huge amounts of poor quality food. The emphasis must be on buying good quality food and not to have second helpings. This does not mean that the food portion must look tiny. On the contrary, studies indicate that the apparent size of a portion plays a significant role in the feeling of fullness regardless of how many calories are actually present. Water already present in food for example in soup or in tomatoes gives a feeling of fullness because it leaves the stomach more slowly than plain water. Air added to whisked eggs makes the portion look bigger. This has given rise to the idea of presenting sensible food as a bigger volume and in a more appetizing fashion. Lots of vegetables and several portions of fruit can add bulk to the meal, be it the main course or dessert, and can fill you up without eating huge portions of fat and sugar. Soup can reduce the amount eaten for the main course.

Reduce the full fat crisps and the fizzy drinks. The excess fat eaten will be deposited as fat and too much carbohydrate will also be converted into fat. Excessive refined carbohydrate (sweet foods like biscuits, cakes and sweets) will add weight so these must not be eaten on a regular basis. Try to buy home-produced food because if food does not have to travel far it should contain fewer chemicals, fewer preservatives and fewer flavour and texture enhancers. Time must be found for preparing a meal containing vegetables every day and fresh fruit of any or every kind should be eaten every day. Small portions of dried fruit can be eaten on occasions as snacks. Fast processed meals must not be consumed on a regular basis. In children regular 'fast food' may lead to lack of attainment of real potential, and to hyperactivity. The often over-heated and over-used oils in fast food are not conducive to good health and may contain cancer-inducing substances.

Medical Organizations have opposed a call from the Business Confederation for the introduction of new health charges for those with lifestyle disorders such as overeating with obesity, however a tax on 'fast foods' has been introduced in some EU countries and in Australia. In common with some British and US airlines Irish carriers may start charging overweight passengers for two seats.

Remember that your own hips are the best that you will ever get, so keep them as long as possible! If you are reasonably thin, stay that way. If your parents were obese resolve not to become obese too, by attention to a sensible diet and exercise. Your GP can be very supportive and even a once yearly weight record will help you to maintain a reasonably stable weight. It is much healthier to keep a stable, even non-ideal weight for height rather than fluctuating above and below that weight. See Table 1.

The bushmen of the Kalahari desert have known for many years that a plant similar to a cactus, called Hoodia gordonii, has the ability to stave off hunger when food is scarce. Commercial development of this product may be feasible and if so it may be a huge step forward for those who crave a safe product that keeps the calories down because the brain tells you that you are not hungry!

In the UK an ant-obesity drug is now available over the counter in pharmacies, for obese people with BMI of 30 or more. This acts by inhibiting the absorption of fat which gets excreted. The subject has to follow a low fat diet and will need adequate vitamin intake to replace the vitamins lost in the fat. Drug companies are also working on the commercial production of a hormone called adiponectin. A hormone is a substance possessing a regulatory effect on the body. Adiponectin is present in the fat cells of our bodies and normally keeps us in shape, however eating the wrong food with weight gain affects and overwhelms its regulatory action. A new drug will soon be available which increases adiponectin and may prove very useful for the treatment of obesity and diabetes and may even prevent the development of full blown diabetes in susceptible individuals. Over the years pharmaceutical companies have produced some great drugs so maybe adiponectin will prove to be the slimming agent of the twenty-first century however it is worth remembering that only one in ten new drugs offer better health treatment. It is also essential to remember that weight loss medications are most effective in association with a sensible diet and increased exercise.

Liposuction is a fashionable and popular treatment for removing unsightly fat. Some fat cells are necessary for all individuals. They have a role in stabilizing metabolism and perhaps may even help prevent type 2 diabetes. Liposuction may in some cases remove this stabilizing force so although the body appearance may improve it may not be the ideal treatment for everyone. Exercise and sensible eating are cheaper and are a wiser way of staying in shape. It is important to keep in mind that while being overweight may affect your looks, that this is not the main reason for losing weight. There must be a sense that regardless of appearance i.e. whether the person is beautiful with or without curves, flesh rolls or a big posterior, that the healthy option is not to damage the heart by asking it to pump blood through excessive fat! The bottom line is "Save your heart and avoid illness and premature death"! You do not want to have your mother or grandmother help you reach the toilet or help you into a wheelchair if you can avoid this by curbing weight gain as soon as possible. If you do not eat one biscuit per day almost 20,000 calories can be removed from the diet per year. Try to adhere to a sensible diet most of the time and have an occasional luxury some of the time. In shops, choose stairs instead of escalators. Take public transport for at least some journeys. Try a different hobby than switching on the TV. Get a dog who will make you thinner, happier and full of vigour and help yourself while reducing the national scandal of putting down millions of healthy dogs.

About 3500 kilocalories of food is equivalent to half a kilogram or 1 pound weight approximately. To lose 1 kilogram a week reduce food intake by about 500 kilocalories per day (3-4 biscuits) and exercise by walking, helping with the vacuuming, mowing the lawn and dancing to music, if possible each for 30 minutes per day! You may not be able to do all of these activities per day but you can try! The first step is to reduce the amount of fat and sugar in the diet. A great first move is to avoid chips and substitute boiled potatoes. Alcohol is high in calories so avoid excess. Low alcohol drinks are not beneficial since these are often high in calories. The secret is to have a small amount of alcohol and supplement with low calorie soft drinks or water. Do not overdo the allowed 2-3 units of alcohol /day.

If you do not want to count calories make a few small changes to start with. Stop the biscuits and cakes on a regular basis and have fruit instead, Do not eat 'seconds'. Take a walk or two or dance to music. Remember any weight loss is a positive effect and the slower it falls off the greater the chance of it staying off!

Losing and gaining weight is not a good idea. It diminishes self-confidence and is unhealthy as the body's metabolism gets all mixed up from a barrage of signals! To avoid this happening try and get a more balanced pattern going, even if it means accepting yourself at a non-ideal but lighter weight. Eat a balanced diet. Avoid too many processed foods. Vary the food and never have too much of anything! Take small amounts of cinnamon and ginger if you get foods containing them. These are anti-cancer and help stimulate weight loss. Do not add too much salt to your meals. Drink as much fluid as you can but do not overdo this. Irish people drink less water than other Europeans even though it is a commodity we should have plenty of! Get plenty of exercise and sleep adequately. Get a hobby and forget about weight by getting interested in other subjects!

Key sentences: Eat a balanced diet. Avoid too many processed foods. Get plenty of exercise and sleep adequately. Get a hobby and forget about weight by getting interested in other subjects!

20

Heart Disease

Cardiovascular disease is the leading cause of death in developed countries. Despite a steady decline in death rates from heart disease, Ireland still has excess mortality compared to most EU countries. There is a higher rate of deaths from heart disease amongst the lower social classes and in the north-east and the south.

The increased prevalence of obesity and diabetes mellitus is now putting men, women and children at risk of heart disease. Body mass index (BMI) adjusts weight for height. Elevated BMI is a risk factor for diabetes and cardiovascular disease, but waist size is a better indicator of risk for both diabetes and heart disease. In the unlikely but possible situation that a man has a waist size greater than 40 inches, or a woman has a waist bigger than 35 inches then both are at risk of heart disease even if they have a normal BMI *. Other major risk factors for heart disease include high blood pressure, cigarette smoking and high blood fat levels. Although there has been a decrease in smoking, rates are still too high amongst young men and women. Cigarette smoking can be stopped with a strong will and if necessary with the help of nicotine patches or specific tablets which your doctor can prescribe. To avoid high blood pressure, BMI must be kept at least below 30, as little salt consumed as possible and alcohol excess avoided. About one in four heart patients has diabetes.

*   *people with BMI greater than 30 must lose at least a few pounds, eat sensibly, leave the car at home and start exercise*

people with BMI between 25 and 29 must not gain any more
weight, and should leave the car at home and start exercise
men and women must keep their waistlines at least below 40
and 35 inches respectively and preferably below 32 and 28
respectively.
BMI is calculated from weight in kg and height in metre. For
example a person of weight 60 kg and height 1.6 metre has a
BMI of 60 divided by 1.6 squared:
=60/2.56 or 23.4
1 pound =0.45 kg and 1 foot = 0.3 metre =30 centimetre

In general, men die twice as often as females from heart disease. In females, oestrogen has a protective effect before the menopause. While oestrogen may protect the blood vessels against the build-up of fatty deposits which increase the risk of heart disease, there is no clear evidence that hormone replacement therapy or the contraceptive pill decrease the risk of heart disease. Women of middle age have a greatly increased risk of dying from a heart attack. One year after a heart attack, 42% of women will have died compared with 24% of men. Women are often treated less urgently and are given less effective treatment than men because of the belief that still exists that a man is far more likely to get a heart attack than a woman.

Diagnosis of a heart attack can sometimes be difficult. Pain affects the sexes differently and they respond differently to analgesics (painkillers). Women may experience a heart attack as diffuse pain in the left shoulder with nausea. Men get central chest pain radiating down the left arm. There are however many other reasons for shoulder, chest and arm pain besides heart disease! If there is a family history of heart disease, see your GP who will measure your blood pressure, organise some blood tests to check your blood fat and blood sugar, and you may also need an electrocardiogram (ECG) taken during controlled exercise. Your GP may prescribe you aspirin as a preventive measure to avoid the stickiness sometimes found in blood. It is important for you to discuss all medication prescribed with your GP to ensure that the benefits of taking this outweigh the risks. Aspirin taken in low dose has a preventive effect against heart disease. In women low dose aspirin may also have a preventive action against the development of stroke. In men the preventive action of aspirin in stroke is not that clear but may be beneficial.

Chest pain brought on by effort, exposure to cold or by anxiety can be due to angina. Cold weather can double the number of heart attacks in those at risk so always wrap up sensibly when walking in cold weather. Do not push a car to start it in cold weather. Use public transport instead. Use the money saved from giving up cigarettes to get an annual car service but avoid using the car excessively.

Take preventive action to avoid heart disease. Anxiety, hostility and depression can cause severe stress and elevation of stress hormones which can cause a heart attack. Get a lifestyle that minimizes the likelihood of clogging the heart arteries. Do not smoke. The car must be left at home as much as possible and physical activity increased by walking at least as far as public transport! Salt must be used sparingly and eat plenty of porridge, fresh fruit and vegetables to increase fibre. Ways of curbing weight gain and adjusting the various types of cholesterol have already been discussed in chapters 3 -6. An LDL-cholesterol reduction of about 35% cuts the risk of heart disease substantially. This is a very good reason for adhering to a sensible diet. If diet fails to stabilize blood fat levels, the fat -lowering drugs called statins may reduce the risk of cardiovascular events including heart attack and stroke but avoid tablets unless you really need them.

Classical music can be very relaxing and may help reduce heart rate and blood pressure. Loud rapid music has the opposite effect however modern music can also be relaxing provided its tempo is smooth and calming. Avoid excessive alcohol. While the recommended amount of alcohol of 21 units per week for men and 14 units for women may be good for your heart, more than this may increase triglyceride fats and blood pressure. If in spite of a sensible diet with reduced salt intake, moderate alcohol and exercise, the blood pressure remains high a small amount of a diuretic, which removes water from the body, may be necessary. Parsley and asparagus are natural diuretics.

Children who eat lots of meals outside the home are likely to face greater heart disease risk factors with higher blood pressure and lower HDL. HDL is the good heart-protecting cholesterol. Habits form early so encourage children to eat sensibly with plenty of fresh fruit and vegetable snacks, and to exercise. Attention to the teeth is also important.

We must take 'heart' from the experience in Finland ! In the seventies, Finland had the highest rate of coronary mortality in the world. A team of health workers set about improving diet with lowering of cholesterol, increasing exercise, reducing smoking and lowering blood pressure by reducing salt intake. Finland today, as a result of these means has reduced obesity and the national rate of mortality from cardiovascular disease has fallen by almost 70%.

Sudden Cardiac Death Syndrome (SCDS) has been diagnosed in several young people, particularly sportsmen, in recent years. In such cases there may be a family problem with the heart muscle or an electrical fault. Everyone should be aware that sudden death in a relative at a relatively young age (< 50 years of age) should be investigated. This is in order to avoid missing a condition that might be diagnosed early and prevented from causing illness or death in relatives of the dead person.

The American Heart Foundation has emphasised the importance of history taking from subjects entering competitive sports. The personal and family history is very important. Examination must include detailed cardiac examination in the supine and standing positions including examination of all pulses and listening for any heart murmurs. Referral to a cardiologist will be necessary if any abnormalities are found. Screening is not easy in the young and despite a normal screening it is impossible to say that an individual will never die from a cardiac event on the sports field, however it is important to remember that SCDS is rare. It is also important to stress the dangers of taking illicit drugs or any form of body-building or sport-enhancing drugs. Cocaine use has been incriminated in sudden death due to a heart muscle abnormality called cardiomyopathy.

Exposure to bacteria and viruses early in life may have an important impact on health affecting the later development of heart disease. The bacterium chlamydia pneumoniae may cause arterial inflammation allowing fatty substances to attach to the arterial walls and eventually allowing arteries to be clogged. A cytomegalovirus may stimulate formation of smooth muscle cells that can cause plaque formation in arteries. Viruses can attack the heart and lead to sudden death. It is important if possible to maintain a healthy immune system by exercise and sensible eating, avoiding smoking and avoiding exposing children to smoke. Do not burn rubbish in the garden. Dioxins and other hazardous fumes may cause health hazards. Avoid slurry pits as these give off fumes which can be toxic to the heart. Any environmental damage may expose you and your family to unhealthy pathogens. Do not consume excess alcohol and never take recreational or performance-enhancing drugs.

Some prescription drugs can affect the heart rhythm and may cause fainting. If a newly prescribed drug is causing any such problems see your GP immediately.

Dublin City Council has introduced automated electronic defibrillators. It is intended that these devices are located so that a victim with a life-threatening cardiac arrhythmia can be treated within 3 minutes. In the future there will be more extensive deployment of automated external defibrillators in railway stations, airports, ferry ports, shopping centres and bus stations. The HSE will devolve responsibility for the defibrillators to the appropriate ambulance services who will also train volunteers to use them appropriately.

Key sentences: A LDL-cholesterol reduction of about 35% cuts the risk of heart disease substantially. Habits form early so encourage children to eat sensibly with plenty of fresh fruit and vegetable snacks, and to exercise. Do not smoke or consume excess alcohol and never take recreational or performance-enhancing drugs.

21

Diabetes Mellitus

In the body, the blood sugar is kept finely balanced by a sugar storage system in the liver and by insulin from the pancreas. Sugar is absorbed by the body's cells through the influence of insulin and used to produce energy. When insulin has done its work it is broken down and therefore supplies of insulin must constantly be renewed. When there is either insufficient insulin or the insulin is not efficient, the blood sugar rises and diabetes is manifest by increased thirst, increased urination, tiredness, blurred vision and in the so-called juvenile or type 1 diabetes there is weight loss.

There are two main types of diabetes-type 1 which occurs mainly but not exclusively in young people and requires insulin for treatment, and type 2 diabetes which used to occur mainly in overweight middle-aged people but is now occurring in teenagers mainly because of obesity. The majority (90%) of cases of diabetes are type 2. Type 2 diabetes affects 2- 6% of the population. Blood sugar testing by pharmacists in Ireland has revealed that about 5% of the people tested had diabetes but were unaware that they had this. These subjects were referred to their GPs for follow-up thus allowing early intervention. At least 6% of people over the age of 65 years have diabetes due to decreased activity.

There may be a link between social class and incidence of diabetes with a lower incidence of diabetes in higher employment grades compared to lower grades. This is probably related to better nutrition, exercise and less smoking in the higher-skilled workers. Exercise even without weight loss can increase the ability of insulin to keep the blood sugar in check. Hereditary factors are important in type 2 and the disease is often triggered by obesity in individuals susceptible to diabetes by virtue of their genes. Although in this type of diabetes there are usually adequate amounts of insulin, the subject is insensitive to the insulin and consequently the blood sugar is elevated. This condition often remains undiagnosed for many years. People likely to be susceptible to diabetes often have a family history of diabetes, are overweight or have a history of diabetes during pregnancy. These individuals should have at least their urine tested for sugar (glucose) or preferably have a fasting or post-meal blood sugar measured. The blood test is the more sensitive test. Subjects with a history of elevated blood pressure, heart disease or blood fat elevation may also become susceptible to diabetes and should have a sugar test. The use of certain drugs including steroids may on occasions make a person susceptible to diabetes.

Type 2 is now common in obese teenagers, something unheard of twenty years ago. Children who eat lots of meals outside the home have been found to have lower sensitivity to insulin making them more vulnerable to get diabetes. They are also likely to face greater heart disease risk factors with higher blood pressure and lower HDL, the heart-protecting cholesterol.

Lack of sleep may increase appetite and has been found to have a disruptive effect on our ability to balance our blood sugars. People who continually get little or too much sleep may be more susceptible to type 2 diabetes. Eight hours give or take an hour seems the desirable sleep time. Smoking increases the risk of getting diabetes by reducing the effect of insulin on glucose control.

Diabetes is at least four times more common in Asians than Europeans. Asian men and women are at greater risk from heart disease than non-Asians. It is essential with our immigrant population that interpreters are present if necessary, to ensure that an adequate history is received from the Asian patient who may on occasions not have enough English to help express his symptoms adequately.

In type 1 diabetes the cells in the pancreas that produce insulin have been destroyed so the blood sugar remains high. Although hereditary factors are linked with this type of diabetes, it is not directly inherited, so environmental factors probably trigger this disease in genetically susceptible individuals. Although type 1 diabetes generally occurs in non-obese subjects, diet may be a triggering factor for this disease. Type 1 diabetes is occurring in younger and younger children and it is possible that twenty-first century diet may have caused the age of incidence to drop. Type 1 is manifest by weight loss, tiredness, frequent urination and thirst. Insulin injections are needed for treatment. Children who have type 1 diabetes are likely to have better blood glucose control if they have a positive attitude and realize that being a diabetic does not bar them from any recreation or sport provided they take suitable precautions with regard to their blood sugar. Adults with type 1 diabetes must also ensure that they are not discriminated against in jobs or in driving because subjects who are stabilised on insulin perform well within almost all employments and have no more road traffic accidents than non-diabetic subjects.

Some experts believe that type 1 diabetes and type 2 diabetes are one and the same disorder with manifestation times being different due to speed of the destruction of the pancreatic β-cells which produce insulin. Lifestyle changes in the past thirty years which have led to obesity and lack of exercise may trigger not just type 2 but also type 1. The role of bacteria and viruses early in life may also have an important impact on health affecting the later development of diabetes. Excessive use of cleaning agents in the home may not allow the immune system to develop to its full potential with exposure to bacteria and viruses early in life possibly having an important impact on health affecting the later development of diabetes. At the time of diabetes manifestation reshuffling of genes may occur with the release of ribonucleic acid (RNA) from previous viral infection and this may trigger a reaction in which the body attacks its own tissues.

In both types of diabetes, poor blood sugar control and smoking can lead to severe eye, kidney or limb complications. Diabetes causes foot ulcers and about 22% of all major amputations. Every minute someone in the world may need a foot amputation because of diabetes. High blood sugars have a negative effect on heart perfusion. Diabetic patients have at least double the risk of heart disease compared to non-diabetic patients and diabetes can affect the heart muscle, the blood vessels and nerves to the heart. Depression is said to be higher amongst diabetic patients compared to the general public. This may be related to blood sugar fluctuation. In the 45-64 age range the risk of death is increased nearly 2-fold compared to non-diabetics. Since heart disease is a major factor in the morbidity of both types of diabetes and inflammation of arteries seems to play a major part, it is important to control not just the diet, exercise and the blood sugar but attention must be paid to avoidance of smoking and good control of blood pressure and blood fats.

Erectile dysfunction occurs in male diabetic patients due to poor circulation to the penile area. As with non-diabetic patients, tablets called phosphodiesterase inhibitors can be used to help this erectile disability. Unfortunately these drugs may not be suitable in all diabetic patients with erectile dysfunction because of disease complications. A sublingual form of tablet may soon become available which would allow the use of a lower dose of the product. This would have a beneficial erectile effect without major side effects. Sublingual means that the tablet dissolves under the tongue. Your GP will be very helpful in deciding the best tablet for you. It is important to have diabetes detected early in order to start treatment as soon as possible. The blood sugar must be well-controlled. In type 2 it is necessary to at least keep the weight from increasing or preferably achieve some weight loss by adherence to diet and exercise. The key to all diet adherence is flexibility. With the great choice of food available today, any diet can be followed and a diabetic diet is a sensible diet that anyone can follow. Type 1 diabetic patients require insulin in addition to diet and exercise. Some patients with type 1 diabetes may have a short interim period following diagnosis, during which their sugars seem to improve spontaneously without the need for insulin. This is called the 'honeymoon' period but usually does not last too long!

Good diabetic control is where blood sugars are kept as close as possible to normal with avoidance of high and low sugars. With good blood sugar control, exercise and absence of smoking, eye, kidney and limb complications arising from diabetes can be significantly reduced and there is recent evidence that heart disease can also be reduced with good diabetic control. There are lots of patients in Europe and in the US who have been on insulin for more than forty years and who have avoided serious eye, kidney, limb and heart complications through good blood sugar and blood pressure control, through exercise and avoidance of obesity and smoking.

Type 2 diabetic patients may require tablets or occasionally, insulin in addition to diet and exercise in order to control their blood sugars, either from time of diagnosis or as time goes by. There are lots of tablets available for control of the blood sugar, some new and some that have been available for many years. Some of these can cause a low blood sugar so it is important if taking these tablets, to be aware of possible interaction with alcohol which can also cause a low blood sugar. One of the older tablets still widely used, is called metformin. This may have an anti-cancer effect as well as a weight reducing effect and its advantage is that it lowers the blood sugar without causing a low blood sugar. A new type of tablet can help smooth out blood sugars after meals. Talk to your GP about this. Insulin is now available by inhaler.

Tablets prescribed for weight loss can help type 2 diabetic patients to lose some weight. Some of these 'slimming' tablets contain a fat enzyme inhibitor. An enzyme is a protein which can speed up or slow down chemical reactions. The enzyme inhibitor causes reduced fat absorption so vitamin supplements would be necessary. Other tablets for weight loss, increase the levels of the hormones noradrenaline and serotonin and speed up metabolism. A hormone is a substance possessing a regulatory effect. Generally the amount of weight loss with these tablets is small and more importantly the long-term health benefits of these drugs remain unclear. Another group of tablets increases the hormone adiponectin which is naturally present in all of us however eating the wrong foods affects and overwhelms its regulatory action. This group may prove useful for the treatment of obesity and diabetes and may even prevent the development of full blown diabetes in susceptible individuals, however the long-term safety of these tablets remains to be seen.

As with all people, exercise is extremely important in everyday life in people with diabetes, who are more at risk than the general population from blood pressure elevation and heart disease. Diabetic blood sugar control is definitely improved following exercise including walking, bicycling and swimming. When tablets are used in type 2 diabetes there are usually few problems with low blood sugars. With insulin, extra care is needed when exercising, to avoid low blood sugars. Depending on the type of exercise, extra calorie intake or insulin dose reduction to suit the particular exercise may be necessary. Exercise-induced low blood sugars are not common in adolescent diabetic patients provided appropriate practical precautions have been taken. If you have diabetes always examine your feet after exercise to ensure that no cuts or bruises have occurred. Remember to take someone with you when going swimming whether you are diabetic or not. Water and sea can be unpredictable!

It is unnecessary and expensive for diabetic subjects to buy low-sugar products such as beans and chocolate. It is important to remember that a diabetic person can eat everything a non-diabetic person eats but that products that raise the blood sugar rapidly must be consumed in small amounts over an extended time period, except of course in a low blood sugar emergency when it is desirable to raise the blood sugar rapidly. Products that raise the blood sugar quickly include for example those containing glucose syrup or sucrose. Those diabetic patients using insulin may need an extra unit or so of insulin if consuming excessive sucrose in say sweets or pastries, which should not occur too frequently to avoid too much weight gain!

Always discuss with your doctor the signs and symptoms of a low blood sugar which can result from taking too many sugar lowering tablets but particularly if you are using insulin. Symptoms often include headache, inability to concentrate, confused behaviour, incoherent speech, blurred vision and fits. Find out what to do if your blood sugar goes down low for example after strenuous exercise when you may not have taken an adequate snack prior to exercise. In an emergency, glucose syrup or a glucose gel can help to stop the onset of a low blood sugar. The glucose is quickly absorbed making it a fast effective source of energy.

If you enjoy alcohol, take it in moderation:

Recommended amounts are 2-3 measures a day for males or 21 measures per week, 1-2 measures for female or 14 measures per week. A measure equals a unit and is equivalent to half a pint of beer, lager or cider or 1 small glass of sherry or of wine or 1 single tot of spirits. One bottle of wine is 7 units.

Never drink alcohol without taking some food as a low blood sugar may result. **Never drink and drive**. Do not smoke.

The fat-lowering drugs called statins (There are several of these) may reduce the risk of cardiovascular events including heart attack and stroke in patients with and without diabetes. Many diabetic patients have elevated LDL-cholesterol (bad cholesterol) and low HDL- cholesterol (good cholesterol) and statins should be used if possible in those patients. Research has also indicated that statins may improve the health and longevity of diabetic patients even if these patients have relatively low LDL- cholesterol levels. Talk to your GP about this.

Diabetes needs regular monitoring. You will be able to test your own blood sugar at home with a glucometer and to bring a record of your sugars to your doctor. It is important to have your doctor test your blood pressure, your blood fats and your urine for micro amounts of protein. A screening test for haemochromatosis should be made as this condition is common in Irish people and it can trigger diabetes. Regular screening for eye problems is essential with full examination at least every 2 years and more frequently if you already have eye complications. Glaucoma is fairly common in diabetic patients and care with the use of eye drops used in the clinic to dilate the pupil is important, as these can trigger glaucoma.

Subjects with diabetes need support and continuous update regarding ways of monitoring their blood sugar. Prisoners with diabetes often have difficulty getting adequate facilities to monitor their blood sugars and may need to get ongoing advice for blood sugar control. A facility should be made available to allow shared care between themselves and their doctors.

In the US, 1 in 20 A & E admissions are said to be due to reactions to tablets. The situation is probably similar in Ireland. Take the medication prescribed by your doctor but always ask your doctor and pharmacist about:

- the dose prescribed

- the side effects both short and long-term

- and if there are alternatives that might suit you better.

There is no reason to think that subjects with high blood pressure, cardiac problems or diabetic patients taking insulin, make a substantial contribution to RTAs however as with all road users, subjects taking tablets or injections must be conversant with the medical aspects of fitness to drive for their own sake and for public safety. If you are taking any tablets or injections it is important to be stabilized on these before driving. Your GP will advise you regarding this and also what you must declare regarding your eyesight and health when applying for a driving licence.

There are many thousands of people who have undetected diabetes. Undetected diabetes is leaving thousands at risk of a heart attack. People susceptible to diabetes mellitus include: obese individuals, those with a family history of diabetes mellitus particularly in first degree relatives like children or brothers or sisters, people with high blood pressure, people with blood fat disorders, people taking certain medication e.g. steroids and women who had diabetes during a pregnancy. If you have a family history of diabetes, have put on weight and are feeling tired with little energy it is important to have at least a urine test but preferably a blood test for diabetes. The number of diabetic patients in the world is set to double by 2010 because of obesity. If we shut off every escalator on earth we could reduce the development of diabetes. There is evidence that in subjects at risk for type 2 diabetes, exercise may act as a preventive measure. Avoid getting diabetes if possible, by exercise and keeping weight as steady and as near to ideal as is practical for you. Do not let your weight keep climbing! Do not smoke.

If you do have diabetes it is important to remember that some world class athletes including footballers have diabetes and are taking insulin. They do not allow their diagnosis or treatment to hinder their sporting achievements. For diabetic subjects taking insulin who are involved in competitive sports the trick is to take adequate snacks or to adjust your insulin if you are doing strenuous exercise. Individuals always work out what suits them and often they can adjust the insulin or diet to a very fine degree. There are many new fast-acting insulins available that will allow you to control your blood sugar very well and avoid low sugar reactions occurring either during or after exercise or during the night following the exercise. Insulin is also available by inhaler. Talk to your GP about these.

Key sentences: Avoid getting diabetes if possible, by exercise and keeping weight as steady and as near to ideal as is practical for you. Do not let your weight keep climbing! If you have a family history of diabetes, have put on weight and are feeling tired with little energy it is important to have at least a urine test but preferably a blood test for diabetes.

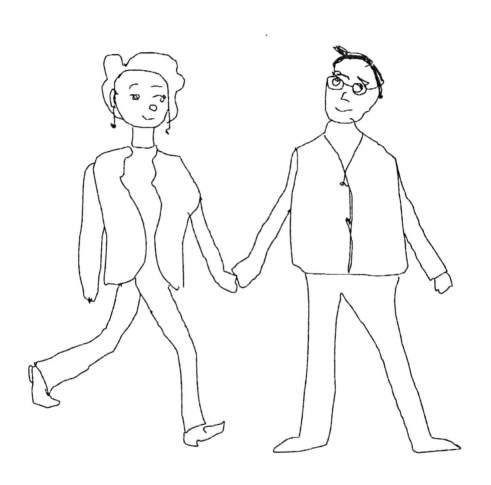

EXERCISE IS THE KEY TO HEALTH PROMOTION

22

The Patient

It is desirable that illness is prevented, however sometimes illness will occur and you may have to call the doctor. Your history is very important. Your race, ancestry and your birthplace can be very informative. Some diseases are much higher in Irish people than in other nationalities e.g. haemochromatosis which is a disorder in which iron is absorbed in excess, and coeliac disease, a small bowel disorder. Multiple sclerosis may also occur more commonly in people from the north of Ireland. Haemochromatosis may initially be manifest by increased pigmentation. People with one gene for the condition are usually carriers for the disease and can pass it on to relatives while those subjects with two genes usually develop the disease. It is more common in 40-60 year old males and in post-menopausal women because pre-menopausal women tend to lose iron during their menstrual periods. If undiagnosed, haemochromatosis can cause heart damage, diabetes, problems with the testes, impotence, cirrhosis, liver cancer and in males, osteoporosis. Treatment involves removing blood on a regular basis until the iron drops to a normal level. It is interesting that iron poisoning has been linked with the occurrence of multiple sclerosis.

Metabolic diseases are also relatively high in the Irish population. If there is a family history of recurrent baby deaths at an early age this should be mentioned to your GP.

Coeliac disease is a disorder of the small bowel caused by a reaction to a protein called gluten which is found in wheat, rye, barley and in oats. Coeliac disease occurs in 1 in 300 people in the west of Ireland whereas it occurs less frequently in other parts of Ireland and in the UK. Coeliac disease can occur in association with diabetes. It can be difficult to diagnose and is often missed because there may be vague symptoms such as chronic fatigue. If the diagnosis is missed which it frequently is, complications such as infertility, calcium deficiency with epileptic fits, osteoporosis and cancer of the small bowel may occur.

Alcoholism is a major problem in Ireland and is a major cause of family disruption. Do not be afraid to seek help for this.

The GP is extremely valuable to children from broken homes or upset by family breakdown.

If you suffer with stammering you may wish to contact the Irish Stammering Association or your GP.

If there is a history of suicide in the family you may wish to join a support group. GROW and STOP are two such groups.

You may have a physical or mental problem or indeed you may not have either but require advice and feel that your GP is the best one to give this. You may have injured yourself playing football. What you tell the doctor gives him the clues needed to find a diagnosis. GPs are often stressed just like anyone else but with the added stress of responsibility for human life. Sometimes therefore the doctor needs as much help as he can get to form a diagnosis! So before you get to the doctor and find yourself unable to explain how you feel some tips are useful. Write down your main complaint and try to describe any problems you think are associated with it:

- What is your main complaint? (for example headache, constipation, vomiting, pain, lack of sex drive, cough)

- When did it commence?

- Where did it start?

- Ever had this type of complaint previously?

- What makes it better or worse? When is it worst?

- Did you take anything for the complaint?

- Are there other associated problems? Can you pass urine? Have you any bowel problems?

- Any weight loss?

- Any bone or muscle pain?

- Any skin rash ?

- Do you feel chronically tired?

- Do you smoke? Do you drink alcohol? Are you taking cocaine or other substances?

- Have you been taking any tablets, injections, herbal remedies or laxatives? Are you using eye drops, a nasal spray or an inhaler?

- Have you had any illnesses or operations in the past?

- Is anybody else in the house sick?

- Are there any illnesses (heart disease, sudden death, or cancer) in the family?

- Have you chest pain, palpitations or a rapid heart beat?

- Did the problem begin after sexual intercourse?

- Have you fainted or had blackouts?

- Have you sudden unexplained shortness of breath?

- Do you live on a farm?

- Have you a pet animal(s) at home?

- Have you been in the country recently ? i.e. up hills, in a forest or wading in water?

- Have you been abroad recently?

- Have you had any vaccinations lately?

- Were there any changes made to the house recently i.e. new paintwork, new central heating etc?

- Do you use pesticides?

- What is your job?

- Are you getting enough sleep?

- Are your menstrual periods regular?

- Are you reasonably happy?

- **Are you allergic to anything?**

Make sure that you mention any weight loss, tiredness, bone or muscle pain or the presence of a skin rash. If you do get a skin rash only when you go out in the sun this is important information for your GP as it may indicate a family condition or that tablets you are taking are not suitable for you. Spotting a skin rash can solve a diagnosis i.e. a condition called Lyme disease that is common in the US and in parts of Europe, can cause pains in joints, stiff neck, muscle tenderness and swelling of lymph nodes however the most characteristic finding is a skin rash which starts as a red raised or flat area which expands into a ring-shape. Always tell your doctor if you have a lump (s) or swelling (s). *Blood* appearing in sputum, vomit, urine or faeces is an immediate signal for consulting your GP.

As a customer or patient you need a sense of control and to achieve better lifestyle and health through empowerment. It is important therefore to keep informed about the common and some uncommon medical conditions below.

Acne often occurs at puberty and is caused by increased sebum secretion from the sebaceous glands, often with blocking of pores. This will improve and often goes away with increasing maturity. Dietary advice with avoidance of chocolate, increased fruit intake and face washing with mild antiseptics often helps. In some cases the acne is severe and can cause undermining of confidence. The GP may need to prescribe antibiotics or refer the young person to a skin specialist.

While figures are not available in Ireland it is thought that 5% of hospital admissions are due to *adverse drug reactions*. It is important to remember that drugs are licensed on the basis of a positive benefit versus some risk, as nothing is without risk. Medications which work very well in most individuals may cause reactions in other people. Interactions between drugs or between a drug and alcohol can cause problems. It is not surprising therefore that drugs of all sorts including licensed, unlicensed, 'over the counter' and herbal medicines can cause illness and death in some people since everyone's genetic makeup is different. It is extremely important to tell your GP if you are not feeling good on the prescribed injection or tablets. Post-marketing surveillance of drugs needs to be improved and everyone should think twice before taking any unnecessary tablets. Always read the label or get someone to read it for you. Never take more tablets than prescribed. Never take anyone else's tablets and make sure that children do not have access to tablets not prescribed for them.

Drugs of any kind including alcohol may alter reaction times while driving. **Never drink and drive.** If you have been treated at a dentist's surgery or as a day-case in hospital make sure that you ask if it is safe for you to drive your car. The time taken to achieve road-worthiness varies widely for different anaesthetics and depends on the dose and individual response.

In diabetic patients taking insulin or tablets, hypoglycaemia may impair tracking ability and the subject may be unaware of the impairment. Never drive until your medication is stabilized.

Drugs for epilepsy need to be carefully controlled because a patient may need a drug combination and all drugs have side effects. The individual response to medication must be considered by doctors when advising controlled epileptic patients who are applying for driving licences. Sometimes prescription errors can be made. In the US recently, confusion arose between a drug for heart disease and a similarly-pronounced drug for epilepsy and migraine. If you suspect that there is something wrong with your prescription see your GP or pharmacist.

The incidence of *asthma and hay-fever* are increasing. These conditions are called atopic diseases and are most often due to allergies to a variety of allergens. Asthma sufferers have more asthmatic attacks during the pollen season. Allergies are now increasing to allergens such as fruit, nuts, drugs and to latex. Latex is present in rubber gloves. Allergy to latex was almost unknown before 1980 whereas, nowadays, almost 8% of health workers appear to suffer with this. The increased allergy rate may perhaps be due to cleaner homes and smaller families. Allergies may also be higher in children born by Caesarean section. Exposure to bacteria and viruses early in life may have an important impact on health and the development of the immune system. Early exposure to allergens or microorganisms may affect whether or not there is a later development of heart disease, diabetes, cancer and allergies. Asthma and allergy seems to have a reduced incidence in farmers and their families, possibly because they are exposed early on in life to many allergens. The message may be to stop using so many disinfectants and cleansers. Another suggestion for the increase in atopic disease is that people who get them may have some alteration in their intestinal micro-flora which are bacteria normally present in the gut. Research is ongoing to see if probiotics, which are orally administered micro-organisms, might help these conditions by readjustment of the intestinal micro-flora. Probiotic yoghurt is available. So far there is no convincing evidence that probiotics can prevent or help the symptoms of asthma or allergic rhinitis however the probiotic concentration reaching the gut may be inadequate rather than ineffective and further studies are needed. Vitamin D may be useful in asthma since it may help the body to react more sensitively to steroids which are used to treat asthma.

One hundred people die annually in Ireland from asthma. Asthmatic attacks are frequently precipitated by laughter possibly due to hyperventilation and may indicate that overall control of the condition is not adequate. Asthma sufferers should be aware that a severe attack requiring immediate attention is present if one is too breathless to talk comfortably, or when the prescribed inhaler does not ease the symptoms. Characteristics of severe persistent asthma include continuous symptoms, limited physical activity, frequent exacerbations and frequent night-time symptoms. People with chronic cough may have a substantially reduced air flow and may understandably become depressed. Inhalers with combination therapy of steroids in low dose and long acting bronchodilators may prove helpful. A good discussion with the GP and the Asthma Society of Ireland booklet may prove particularly useful for parents of small children with asthma.

The H5N1 strain *of Avian flu* has killed over 100 people and many millions of birds worldwide. Recently the death of 6 members of the same family in Indonesia has raised fears that bird flu is spreading from person to person. The organism responsible had not mutated and authorities apparently do not know where the infection came from but assume it came from the local poultry market. One key measure to stop avian flu is to keep the birds in more humane surroundings and avoid the gross unhygienic conditions in which they are trapped in many countries. If travelling overseas be wary of overcrowded areas and markets.

Cancer of the bowel is preventable if detected early enough. A sustained change of bowel habit such as diarrhoea or constipation that cannot be explained by eating or drinking something that does not suit you, may be a sign that something is not right with the bowel. You must see your GP who will organise further tests.

Carbon monoxide poisoning still occurs. This may present as headache, tiredness or vomiting. Always make sure that heating devices are in good working order with no condensation or blackening around the appliance, and serviced by a reputable company. If you and the family have symptoms every time that the central heating is turned on, call the servicing company. Acute carbon monoxide poisoning can cause death and chronic carbon monoxide poisoning can lead to neurological conditions such as Parkinson's disease.

Carpal tunnel syndrome is a common condition particularly in women after the menopause and in pregnancy where there are wide fluctuations of hormones. It may also occur in other conditions of abnormal hormone levels such as underactive thyroid and in rheumatoid arthritis. The median nerve is affected in a tunnel of vessels at the wrist, causing numbness and tingling in the hand and fingers, usually sparing the little finger. It tends to go away after the pregnancy is completed. It is helped by avoiding heavy bedclothes and excessive heat. A cortisone injection is often curative. Surgery to relieve the pressure on the nerve is very helpful and is required in severe cases.

Around 1 in 10 children suffer with *constipation*. A good intake of fruit, vegetables and porridge should solve this situation. If necessary a medication for constipation which is not absorbed from the gut and carries water with it, should improve matters. If the constipation continues, further investigation may be needed.

Chronic bronchitis is a lung condition where repeated infections of the airways eventually cause permanent damage leading to a persistent cough and shortness of breath. This can result in pneumonia, emphysema and even heart failure. In emphysema the delicate lung alveoli have lost their elasticity and are badly damaged. Treatment involves stopping smoking, avoiding pollutants and the treatment of infection, however limited lung and heart reserves will limit exercise tolerance. In the past, with the high level of pollutants from coal fires, industry and smoking, large numbers of people were severely incapacitated through ignorance and poor environmental control. In 2006 however it is important that such an outcome is prevented by knowledge and avoidance of smoking, dioxins and other pollutants.

Do not burn rubbish in your back garden.

Contact dermatitis is skin inflammation caused by an allergic or irritating reaction to a product which has been used topically on the body but not necessarily at the area of the skin rash. The use of this agent must stop to prevent further skin inflammation. Lauryl sulphate used in shampoos is a fairly common offender.

Along with the usual precautions, particular caution must be exercised in the prescription of the *contraceptive pill* to smokers or women with a family history of clotting problems.

Deep venous thrombosis (DVT) usually means a clot in the calf veins of the leg. It can cause discomfort or leg pain but the danger lies in the possibility that the clot can be dislodged and go into the lungs. When clots are sent into the lungs, dizziness and nausea or a fainting sensation while sitting in a restricted position or on the toilet may be felt, or sudden death can occur. DVT can affect anyone, particularly the bed-ridden and sick individual. Women who have recently given birth are also at risk of DVT. However it can also affect those who remain immobile for long periods of time when travelling, particularly by plane. Short journeys can also cause DVT if one is taking the contraceptive pill, drinks excessive alcohol and not enough water and is immobile without moving the legs and feet. Never cross your legs while travelling, drink plenty of water with little alcohol and move around if possible or at least move your legs and feet by appropriate exercise. If your leg or foot has been put in plaster make sure to move as much as you can manage and always move the toes. Treatment of DVT involves giving anticoagulants for periods of 3-6 months. These need to be monitored on a regular basis to keep the dose sufficiently high to avoid further clots forming but not so high as to cause bleeding. A device to monitor clotting times at home is now available. Recent research has indicated that DVT can be triggered by infection.

A *dental* visit is periodically worthwhile to ensure that no dental decay or oral problems are present. There has been an increase in recent years in cancer of the mouth in young women. The cause of this is thought to be due to excess alcohol, particularly binge drinking because alcohol can become more concentrated in females because of their smaller body size. There may also be a connection with oral sex. Dentists have detected almost two thirds of these oral cancers. The dentist will give you a form to fill which enquires about any illnesses or medication. *Always tell the dentist if you are taking any form of tablet or injection and if you ever had any illness or allergy*.

Diverticular disease is a relatively common bowel disease which affects 1 in 3 people over the age of 60 years and is often the result of lack of fibre in the diet. The wall of the large bowel contracts quite vigorously trying to compensate for the lack of fibre in the stool and pouches form along the length of the large bowel. The large bowel is a continuation of the small bowel which itself follows on from the duodenum and stomach. The duodenum is a pipe -like area at the end of the stomach. The appendix is between the small and large bowel. The large bowel or colon continues on into the rectum or back passage and anus. The anus is the opening at the end through which waste matter passes out of the body. Inflammation of the pouches causes diverticulitis which often presents itself as pain, fever and nausea. Diverticulitis can be diagnosed by passing a scope into the bowel and viewing the bowel lining, and by X-ray imaging techniques. The condition is helped considerably by increasing the fibre content of the diet by porridge, fruit and vegetables. Diverticulitis is not a malignant condition however diverticulitis and cancer of the bowel can occur together.

The *eye* lens focuses the light, the iris acts like a shutter controlling the amount of light and the image is focused on the retina which sends messages to the brain for interpretation. In long or short sightedness the image is focused in front or behind the retina instead of on it. In astigmatism there is a blurred image because only some of the light is focused. All three conditions can be corrected by appropriate lenses. Retinitis pigmentosa and macular degeneration are two serious eye diseases where recent research has given hope to subjects with these conditions. A microchip implanted in the retina may allow bypass of damaged light-sensitive retinal cells while stimulating other retinal cells and sending impulses to the brain.

Failure to ovulate is a cause of infertility. The pituitary and the hypothalamus are glands in the head which regulate hormonal function. Ovulation failure may be due to problems with either or both glands or due to polycystic ovary syndrome (PCOS). PCOS is due to suppression of the pituitary hormone which regulates ovulation. It causes absence of periods in approximately 7% of pre-menstrual women. It may be found in families and usually starts at puberty. It can cause acne, hirsutism which is excessive hair growth on the face and body, and infertility. Obesity is often present. In PCOS, insulin is secreted in excess although this does not cause a low blood sugar because the body is resistant to its effect. Diabetes may also occur. Male hormones (androgens) are secreted in excess from the ovary probably because of the excess stimulation by insulin. The androgens cause the excessive hair growth. There are quite a few therapies available for PCOS including an anti-diabetic drug which makes the body more sensitive to insulin and which may also help with weight loss. Anti-androgen tablets help the hirsutism and steroids may be used to help with infertility. It is important to be aware that pregnancy can occur while the subject is being treated with steroids.

A *faint* (occurs while the person is standing up) caused by pain or stress can lead to a temporary loss of consciousness. Recovery usually takes place within a couple of minutes because when the person falls, consciousness is restored by blood flowing back towards the heart. If recovery is not rapid, medical attention should be sought.

Common *fungal skin rashes* include athlete's foot presenting with scaling and itching between the toes particularly in hot weather and fungal nail infections which leave the nail thickened, discoloured and fragmented and may also cause a scaly rash between the toes or on the soles of the feet. Ringworm presents as a scaly ring on the body or scalp. Eczema which is not a fungal infection can look very similar to this and diagnosis will have to be confirmed by taking samples of the rash for examination. Candida infection between and under the breasts can cause great discomfort particularly in the obese or elderly. Candida can also cause swelling at the base of the finger nails in subjects who frequently immerse their fingers in water. Patchy loss of pigment on the body after a holiday overseas may be due to a fungal infection on the skin. While none of these infections are life threatening, except in individuals who are immune suppressed due to some other illness, it is important to have them treated for cosmetic reasons, to avoid transmission to other people and to avoid loss of work time. A topical antifungal treatment is very effective. To avoid recurrence some people may have to change work practices.

Haemorrhoids or piles are dilated veins rather like varicose veins, in the rectum and anus. Approximately 1 in 4 people may suffer with these and they can be very painful. Bleeding on passing a bowel movement is often seen as a bright red streak on the toilet paper. Itching and pain are also often present. Pregnant women may get these so prevention is important. To prevent piles occurring, eat porridge, fruit and vegetables on a regular basis and avoid straining to pass faeces or standing for prolonged periods. If you have them, see your GP. Some topical creams may help while the diet is being readjusted however other treatment including surgery may be necessary in advanced cases.

Hay-fever with red eyes and nasal stuffiness can lead to unpleasant symptoms due to over-reaction to allergens. Hay-fever causes a streaming nose, sneezing, red and itchy eyes and nose. Hay-fever is often called rhinitis and is most often due to allergies to a variety of allergens including pollens, grasses and fungal spores. Perennial rhinitis can occur all the year round. Hay fever often begins in the teens but lots of people outgrow it as the immune system matures. Fungal spores may cause symptoms in winter while tree pollens are responsible for at least a quarter of hay-fever cases in spring with grass pollen active in summer. Certain foods such as olive oil and pregnancy can exacerbate hay-fever while other foods such as eggs, milk, oily fish, yoghurt, wholegrains and vegetables may improve symptoms. To help symptoms during a high pollen count keep exposure to a minimum by wearing sunglasses, drying clothes inside, taking a shower after being outside and keeping the car windows shut if possible. Avoid exposure to tobacco smoke, exhaust fumes and perfume which can make the hay-fever worse. To ease nasal stuffiness it is helpful to use a bowl of steaming water containing eucalyptus or menthol drops. If all these measures fail to improve symptoms it may be necessary to get a low-dose steroid nasal spray or non-drowsy forming antihistamine medication.

Some people get rhinitis due apparently to stress and this is called vasomotor rhinitis. People with allergies are more prone than non-allergy sufferers to an uncommon condition called *keratoconus*. This causes the cornea in the eye to become cone shaped rather than the normal curve. Vision becomes blurred. The condition is usually manifest in the late teens but it can be diagnosed at any age. Glasses or contact lenses may help but eye surgery may become necessary.

Headache is a common complaint and is usually not serious, however it can lead to disability and absence from work. There are many causes including, 'tension-type' headache, sinus headache, migraine and a form of migraine called 'cluster headache'. Accurate diagnosis and appropriate treatment of 'cluster headache' are essential because of the intense debility caused by the condition which is more common in men. New research has indicated that a scalp steroid injection may be very helpful in this condition causing long remissions from pain. Migraine can be very disabling, it is relatively common and manifests itself as a one sided throbbing headache that occurs every so often and lasts between 4 and 72 hours. There may be nausea, flashing lights, zig-zag patterns or a tingling feeling in the face or limbs. Dehydration, hunger or disturbed sleep can trigger migraine. Treatment should begin as soon as possible after the start of the pain. There are many treatments available including an over-the- counter treatment soon to become available which contains feverfew and ginger ingredients. Recent research indicates that a small proportion of patients who experience frequent migraine with visual or neurological features, may have a heart defect which can be treated. Dehydration must be avoided in everyone. Ensure that you drink a couple of glasses of water with main meals. Eat some fresh fruit and vegetable daily. Aerosols may cause headache and depression since they emit volatile organic compounds so do not drench the house with aerosols to cover up cooking or smoking smells. People who take drugs for pain on a regular basis may get a so-called analgesic ('painkiller') headache so unless there is a medical condition requiring them, tablets for pain should not be taken on a daily basis.

Headache can on rare occasions be due to meningitis or a brain tumour. Children and adolescents may get headache for a variety of reasons which must be evaluated. High blood pressure does not cause headache. Your history and description will alert your GP to the cause of your headache, the need for further tests and treatment. If regular headache begins after the age of 50 it should be investigated as soon as possible.

Hepatitis B is an infection transmitted through contaminated blood, by sexual intercourse or after tattoos or ear piercing in places with poor hygiene controls. Drug users are often at risk of this infection through the use of contaminated needles. It causes inflammation of the liver which can lead in some cases to long-term chronic infection. Chronic infection with hepatitis B can lead to hepatitis, cirrhosis and liver cancer. Treatment is available for those subjects with chronic infection. Women can infect their children and a considerable proportion of those that become chronically infected are infants or children. Pregnant women should be screened for hepatitis B in order to protect the newborn baby with appropriate treatment including vaccination.

Hepatitis C is a blood-borne infection most often associated with drug users. It can be acquired by blood transfusion or organ transplantation when hepatitis C has not been detected on screening. It can also be acquired on sexual contact or after tattoos or ear piercing in places with poor hygiene controls. The risk of sexual transmission increases if the infected individual has multiple partners. Treatment and follow-up for this condition is available. If in the past you injected drugs and now worry that you may have contracted hepatitis C, a blood test can detect if you have ever been infected or if you need follow-up. Do not feel embarrassed about your past behaviour. You will find that your GP will listen to you sympathetically and may advise testing for your own peace of mind.

A *hernia* occurs when part of an internal organ bulges through muscles into a neighbouring cavity. It may only be manifest as a bulge when a person stands up and disappears on lying down. You should discuss any lumps or bulges with your doctor.

Hirsutism is excessive facial or body hair growth which can cause physical and psychological problems, usually in women. Excessive hair growth in women can be desirable in many cultures however in Northern Europeans and in American countries it is less acceptable. Our genes and race determine hair growth and in all females, hormonal changes at sexual maturity, during pregnancy and during the menopause can increase hair growth. This usually requires no treatment. In fact, if the increased hair growth at puberty is removed it may be stimulated to form a deep growth requiring regular treatment by electrolysis. Sometimes hair growth on the face and body is excessive and unacceptable and creams or electrolysis have to be used. Electrolysis is performed by passing a small electric current to the root of the hair follicle. This must be done with care to prevent scarring. Hirsutism may sometimes be a cause of serious hormonal imbalance when it will need special investigation.

Influenza ('flu') is caused by a virus which changes yearly, so vaccination of vulnerable groups such as the older age group and subjects with diabetes, needs to be given every year.

Irritable bowel syndrome (IBS) is a common bowel condition which causes considerable disability and absence from work. It is manifest by bloating, abdominal pain and episodes of either diarrhoea or constipation. It usually affects females less than 45 years of age. There is no weight loss and appetite is usually normal. The cause of the syndrome is not known but there may be a psychological element precipitated by stress. Certain foods may trigger IBS. These include coffee, processed foods with sugar and unhealthy fats. IBS may also be triggered by antibiotics. IBS is not a malignant condition however IBS and cancer of the bowel can occur together. The diagnosis of IBS is made by exclusion of other diseases including bowel cancer and diverticulitis. IBS is often helped considerably by excluding any food that is thought to trigger the condition such as coffee, sugar-increased foods, and by increasing the fibre content of the diet with porridge, fruit and vegetables. Crystallised ginger in small amounts can also be helpful.

Lactose intolerance is a disorder in which unpleasant stomach or bowel symptoms are experienced as a result of taking milk or dairy products. There is no correlation between symptoms and the amount of product taken. This intolerance may affect a significant proportion of the population and is very common in Asian populations. Subjects may be born with it, may acquire it or it may be secondary to another bowel problem such as coeliac disease. Symptoms of lactose intolerance include abdominal pain, bloating, diarrhoea and in fact are very similar to the IBS syndrome above. Proper diagnosis must be made because once it is confirmed lactose-free products should be used. A soya substitute can be used. Calcium and vitamin supplements may also have to be taken. If soya milk is given to babies make sure that it is full formula. A list of milk-free products can be obtained from the local hospital dietician. Many people with lactose intolerance can eat goat's cheese whereas they cannot eat normal dairy produce.

Legionella is a bacterium which causes Legionnaires' disease and severe pneumonia. The bug whose natural habitat is water, may be acquired accidentally in air conditioning systems or hot tubs. Proper cleaning using a mask over the mouth and nose and gloves, and monitoring of these systems are essential. Legionella is not transmitted from person to person.

Major tranquillisers are used for serious psychiatric conditions, manic depression or severe agitation.

Meningitis is an infection of the covering of the brain and can be caused by a virus or a bacterium. It is important to remember that it is relatively rare. Bacterial meningitis can affect anyone particularly the young adult, children and the elderly. Initial symptoms of meningitis may be non-specific and similar to flu with fever and restlessness. Anyone may become seriously ill within hours with severe headache, vomiting, neck stiffness, tendency to avoid the light, muscle pain, fever, confusion and drowsiness. In children attempts to touch the forehead with their knees causes discomfort. A rash is not always present but if it is visible it will not fade when a drinking glass is pressed against it. Rarely, meningitis can present with large purple blotches on the body and abdominal pain. Severe headache and neck stiffness should always be investigated immediately. Bacterial meningitis can be caused by several bacteria with meningococci B and C, organisms that normally live in the throat or nose being the most common. Vaccination against meningitis type C (and type A) is available. Meningitis C vaccine is given routinely to vulnerable age groups and the incidence of meningitis due to C is decreasing with one death recorded in Ireland in 2004, a big decrease from previous years. Figures have shown that meningitis due to the B organism increased by 50% in 2003 compared to 2002. A vaccine is not yet routinely available for subgroup B but will be, in the near future. Bacterial meningitis can also be caused by the pneumococcus organism which causes pneumonia, and by tuberculosis. Vaccination against both of these organisms is available.

In babies a high-pitched moaning cry, difficulty in waking up, stiffness with jerky movements and rapid difficult breathing can be signs of meningitis. A rash may not always be present. If you feel that your child is not his usual self or that your own headache is not just any headache you may be right! If in doubt consult your doctor immediately.

People travelling to Mecca should discuss prophylactic vaccination against other organisms that can cause meningitis, with their GP.

There are no vaccinations available for viral meningitis but this type is usually less serious than bacterial meningitis. Viruses can however cause encephalitis which can have similar symptoms to meningitis and needs immediate attention.

Multiple sclerosis (MS) is a condition which affects the fat or myelin in the nervous system. There are approximately 5000 subjects in Ireland with the condition. which is twice as common in women as in men. The diagnosis may be difficult initially when a patient complains of a variety of nervous symptoms which on occasions cannot be confirmed by physical examination. New research indicates that early treatment with a drug containing a naturally occurring substance produced by the immune system, can be beneficial. A form of cannabis although not licensed in Europe may also be beneficial for MS patients and may be used at the doctor's discretion. Cannabis itself can cause many health problems and should never be taken for recreational purposes.

Muscle cramp is a painful muscle spasm which is usually short-lived. The affected muscle can be massaged with the fingers until the pain subsides. If the cramp continues, see your GP.

The diagnosis of m*yalgic encephalomyelitis (ME) or chronic fatigue syndrome (CFS)* is often looked upon with suspicion. There is now some research evidence to show that ME may be an organic illness with physiological effects. There may be altered gene expression and abnormalities in the white blood cells of subjects diagnosed with ME. The results could lead to a specific diagnostic blood test and possibly to drug treatment. A drug used to treat herpes infections has recently been found to help symptoms in subjects with ME syndrome, suggesting that a herpes infection may have a role in this condition.

Osteoporosis usually occurs in females when oestrogen levels tend to wane. It may also occur in males who have low levels of testosterone, who abuse alcohol or who are taking steroids.

The risk factors for osteoporosis include:

- a family history of osteoporosis,

- female sex and usually thin build,

- increasing age, postmenopausal woman, poor diet,

- history of an eating disorder,

- use of steroids,

- no exercise,

- smoking and alcohol excess.

Osteoporosis leads to reduced bone strength and an increase in fracture risk. 20% of Irish people who break their hip are at risk of death within 6-12 months of the fall because of immobility, infection and blood clots. It is always best to prevent osteoporosis by avoiding risk factors. The key to osteoporosis prevention is a good well-balanced calcium-containing diet (dairy food in moderation) and exercise with avoidance of smoking and excess alcohol. There are now many new drugs available which can be helpful in the established disease. A rub-on ointment based on nitroglycerine is also being evaluated as a potential treatment for osteoporosis.

Pernicious anaemia is due to vitamin B_{12} deficiency and is relatively common in Irish people. Symptoms may include tiredness, breathlessness and rapid heart beat on exertion. It gives rise to fewer but bigger red cells than normal. A simple blood test will show if you have this. When testing for B_{12} it is also important to test for folic acid as well, since deficiency of B_{12} may be masked if folic acid is taken without adequate supplementation with B_{12}. Pernicious anaemia needs to be treated by injection of the B_{12} vitamin since people with the condition lack a substance called 'intrinsic factor' which normally allows B_{12} to be absorbed from the gut.

Psoriasis is due to a problem with the immune system which causes the skin cells to renew themselves too frequently. Sometimes psoriasis can resemble fungal infections. The commonest type is plaque psoriasis. Stress may precipitate the condition which often occurs in families. Lithium, a drug used to treat manic–depression can also exacerbate psoriasis. Various creams containing small amounts of coal tar or containing vitamin D and steroids can keep the condition under control. For more severe cases, drugs which target the immune system or phototherapy for a limited period can be helpful. Caution with the immune-modulating drugs is advised however because their long-term safety has not yet been established.

Puberty or sexual maturation is a period of emotional and physical change. At this time parental guidance and sensitivity is all-important. Occasionally, when physical development or growth seems abnormal, GP guidance will be necessary. Menstrual period pain is usually self-limiting however it can also be a cause of disability and absence from work. Adequate fluid should be taken in the weeks prior to the event and some non-steroidal anti-pain tablets may also be necessary during the event. Absence of periods can be psychological, caused by weight loss and exercise, chronic illness or by disorders of the ovaries or of the brain. Anti-psychotic drugs may also cause irregularity. Should periods either not commence or become irregular a visit to the GP will be required.

Restless legs syndrome causes uncomfortable tingling and burning in the feet. It may disrupt sleep. It is thought to be due to a lack of dopamine and may be an inherited condition. Dopamine is a neurotransmitter which transmits signals between brain cells and activates smooth muscle. Subjects with this discomfort should be checked for iron deficiency and diabetes. If no abnormalities are found then a few simple measures may cure the problem. Go to bed a little later than usual, avoid stimulants such as coffee or alcohol before bedtime and have a well-balanced diet. In very severe cases drugs used to treat Parkinson's disease may be helpful however the side effects of these drugs may preclude their prescription for otherwise healthy people.

Rosacea is a skin condition which occurs particularly in 30-50 year old females and which can cause redness and spots on the cheeks, nose, chin and forehead. In long-term cases, especially in men, the nose may enlarge. It often clears up spontaneously but topical or oral antibiotics usually taken for six weeks, can be very helpful to clear the spots. Further courses of antibiotics may be necessary if the rash reappears. It is wise to make a list of the agents such as sunlight, foods or environmental agents which aggravate the rash and avoid these. Avoid extreme temperatures, alcohol, stress, spicy food and hot drinks.

Scleroderma is an autoimmune condition which affects many body systems. Autoimmune means that the body reacts against itself perhaps due to early immaturity of the immune system. Scleroderma can sometimes accompany a condition called Raynaud's disease which is a circulatory condition affecting the hands, however most people with Raynaud's disease do not get scleroderma. In scleroderma the fingers may get stiff and the skin may appear shiny, puffy and thickened. There is an Irish Raynaud's and Scleroderma Society from which a booklet on the condition can be obtained.

Scoliosis is a twisting of the spine which often can be corrected by surgery in childhood.

Sinusitis usually refers to either viral or bacterial infection or an allergy of the maxillary sinuses. The inflammation can cause pain along the cheek bones or on the forehead. Inhaling stem from warm water containing a mixture of clove and eucalyptus oil may be extremely useful however an antibiotic may be needed if there is bacterial infection. In severe cases, surgical draining of the sinuses may be necessary.

90% of *skin cancer* in Ireland is preventable. Avoid getting skin cancer by appropriate attention to your skin which in Irish people is very sun-sensitive. A small amount of sun helps the skin to form vitamin D however the continuous exposure of unprotected skin to the sun is not a good idea. Excessive sunlight harms the skin and the eyes. Sunglasses and a wide-brimmed hat can decrease eye exposure to sun by 50%. Never go out in the sun or let any family member go out in the sun without appropriate sunscreen and if necessary use a hat. Never let your children get tanned on a sun-bed. If a spot or mole becomes itchy, gets bigger or starts to bleed see your GP immediately. Moles on exposed areas like the face and hands deserve particular attention. A device that can scan the deep layers of the skin can help improve the detection of malignant melanoma cancer which can as its name implies, be deadly. Pronged exposure to winter sun can be just as damaging as the effects of summer sun.

Sometimes people who are tense, with difficulty *sleeping*, are prescribed tranquillisers. Minor tranquillisers are used for promoting sleep and can be short, medium or long-acting. The short-acting ones are the most likely to produce withdrawal reactions. The use of tranquillisers is often a source of concern to both doctors and patients because of the possibility of dependence. The best way to avoid dependence on tranquillisers is to take them for as short a period as possible- about 4 weeks. There are effective ways of weaning patients off these medications. If you have such a problem your GP will advise you. Exercise taken several hours before bedtime is a more practical and cheaper way of inducing restful sleep than taking tranquillisers. In addition it is important to establish a routine time of going to bed and of getting up. You will be surprised how your own internal clock will wake you at a certain time every morning! Try to adhere to routine even on holidays. It is also important to avoid food, tea, coffee or alcohol near bedtime. Try not to drink too much water near bedtime as getting up to go to the lavatory disrupts the sleep pattern. Obstructive sleep apnoea occurs in middle-aged overweight men and in post-menopausal women. Subjects experience excessive daytime sleepiness because sleep is disturbed by intermittent shutting off of the airway. These subjects have an increased risk of road traffic accidents, heart disease, high blood pressure and of stroke. Treatment for this condition involves losing weight and using a 'continuous positive airway pressure'. This is achieved by wearing a close-fitting mask over the nose and mouth while sleeping and a small air compressor forces air gently into the airways to keep them open. A high-tech pillow, now licensed in the US, that pumps air into the mouth and is powered by a high-strength rechargeable battery may be an alternative treatment.

Snoring may cause significant sleep disruption to a partner. Snoring often occurs in overweight individuals. Simple measures to help the problem include losing at least some weight, a brisk walk several hours before bedtime, avoiding alcohol or tranquillisers before bedtime and not sleeping on one's back. If these measures do not help it is essential to establish that there is not a serious medical reason for the snoring.

More than 8,000 acute *stroke* patients are admitted annually to hospital in Ireland. A BMI of greater than 30 kg/m^2 increases the risk of stroke. Strokes can be avoided by identifying risks such as excess weight, diabetes, high blood pressure or an irregular heart beat, and making simple lifestyle changes by exercising, not smoking, avoiding excess salt and excess alcohol and sensible eating. While aspirin is useful in preventing stroke in women the picture is not that clear-cut in men. It is prudent to use low dose enteric-coated aspirin as a preventive measure where possible. High blood pressure must be treated with a reduced salt intake, avoidance of excess alcohol and if necessary a blood pressure lowering tablet. Tablets called diuretics, which increase urine secretion, are useful in low dose and are probably still the most practical choice, at least initially, in lowering blood pressure in the majority of subjects.

Sudden death is usually due to heart disease. If there is a history of sudden death in you family do go and see your GP. If your relative was over 50 it is likely that he had heart disease due to clogged arteries. Your GP will check your blood pressure, urine or blood sugar (blood sugar is the more sensitive test) and the blood fats. He will also suggest ways of keeping you healthy such as not smoking, keeping steady weight by sensible eating, avoidance of excess salt and of excess alcohol, and exercise. He may also prescribe some aspirin. If your relative was less than 35 when he died there may be a family problem with the heart muscle or an electrical fault. Your GP will suggest what investigations can be done to try and exclude a similar condition in other family members.

If you have a problem with really excessive *sweating* and all the usual remedies have been tried (Tablets called ßeta-blockers may be useful), then your GP may need to discuss further options with you such as a sympathectomy. The sympathetic nervous system stimulates the sweat glands to secrete sweat. These nerves can be selectively cut to prevent over-sweating.

Systemic lupus erythematosus (SLE) is an autoimmune condition, commoner in females than in males, where the body produces antibodies that attack its own tissues. It is a chronic and relapsing condition affecting most body tissues but usually not all at the same time. The commonest symptoms include weakness, painful joints, fever and rashes particularly on the face. The condition can also be triggered by some drugs used to treat other conditions like tuberculosis. Treatment can vary from simple painkillers to corticosteroids or new therapies which treat the immune system. The prognosis for long symptom-free periods is nowadays quite good although the long-term safety of the immune system drugs has not yet been established.

Tuberculosis (TB) has in the past been relatively common in Ireland. Tuberculosis is recurring in Ireland in certain areas where pockets of infection have been found. Many recent cases have been detected, particularly in young men, possibly because of their increased susceptibility due to close contact with carriers, poor diet and excess alcohol intake. World-wide, 3 million people die yearly from TB. Many patients who recover can relapse in the future. TB which may prove resistant to drugs, can occur in patients who have immunosuppression due to AIDS. TB can cause problems in a lot of body organs but particularly in the lungs, in the brain and its coverings causing meningitis or abscess, in the bones and in the kidney. TB is spread by the coughs or sneezes of an infected person but it is usually passed on only after sustained contact. Main symptoms include fever and night sweats, persistent cough, extreme fatigue, shortness of breath, weight loss and later coughing up blood. If these symptoms are present a chest X-ray and skin test will be needed. Before doing the skin test it is important to know if there is any history of previous vaccination against TB. BCG

(Bacille Calmette-Guérin) is a modified strain of bovine tubercle bacillus used for TB vaccination. Vigilance is always needed to ensure that TB does not recur in the community as it can be silent for some time before it is diagnosed!

In Ireland, BCG vaccination is given routinely in most parts of the country, in order to prevent TB infection. Although vaccination is not 100% effective, TB rates have been shown to be higher in areas not practising BCG immunisation. The optimum age for BCG vaccination is at birth. BCG at birth has the advantage that it should not interfere with skin tests used to trace disease contacts. Testing of the sputum for TB has traditionally taken almost 2 months, since the growth of the organism in culture is slow. Quicker ways of testing are now being developed. In addition a new vaccine may become available in the near future which when given with anti-TB drugs can accelerate recovery and protect against re-infection.

You may need certain *vaccinations* depending on your employment (hepatitis B vaccination for those at risk of infection with blood or contaminated syringes), age (flu vaccine in the elderly), state of health (diabetics and those subjects who have had their spleen removed, require certain vaccines). Ask your GP about all vaccination necessary if you intend to travel abroad. If you travel to a hot climate watch out for insect bites, too much sun and loosing too much fluid. You may need an insect-repellant spray or cream on exposed surfaces, a hat, sunblock and bottled water. If you are travelling to an area where malaria is prevalent you will need to take prophylactic tablets. *Two deaths due to malaria, occurred recently in the UK because travellers omitted to take prophylactic tablets.* Vaccines, like drugs can, in certain individuals cause side effects such as muscle weakness or general weakness. It must be emphasised however that in general the benefit of vaccination far outweighs its risks. *Live vaccines should not be given to pregnant or immunocompromised individuals.*

Whooping cough caused by the organism Bordatella pertussis is rising amongst adolescents and adults. This can lead to a severe paroxysmal cough. In addition there is a risk that adults may transmit the infection to infants who may not have been immunised against this organism.

A booster vaccination should be available for adolescents in the near future, making 'herd' immunity more widespread.

Worms can be transmitted from people or can be transmitted by infected meat. Children can get threadworms which are fairly easily treated however with rapid air travel and a multicultural mix of different ethnic groups, more serious worm infestations can arise. Fatal infections may be caused by hookworms in subjects with depressed immunity. Everyone must wash their hands after going to the lavatory. Always buy meat from reputable sources and always cook it fully. Eating 'rare' steaks may not be a good idea.

Acupuncture

The ancient Chinese believed that to be healthy a balance had to be achieved between Yin representing 'quiet' substances and Yang representing 'noise'. Acupuncture particularly for pain does seem to have a validated scientific basis. The Traditional Chinese medicine is symbolised by acupuncture points and channels connecting them. The Gate theory indicates that there is a balance between stimulation of pain fibres and inhibition of the stimulus. Acupuncture stimulates the inhibitory nerve fibres. Acupuncture is now quite widely practised in the US and Europe. It is a medical system that may be of benefit to a patient particularly for pain but should be seen as complimentary rather than an alternative to Western style orthodox medicine. If you need help as to whether or not acupuncture may help you, talk to your GP.

Key sentence: Your history is very important. Your race, ancestry and your birthplace can be very informative. Some diseases are much higher in Irish people than in other nationalities. As a customer or patient you need a sense of control and to achieve better lifestyle and health through empowerment.

23

Men's Health

Men often seem somewhat complacent about their health however it is clear from the male suicide figures in Ireland that many men often suffer from stress while projecting a calm exterior. Men in fact may be just as concerned as women about their health but may also think that it is unmanly to discuss their fears with family or professionals. Although the male brain may react slightly quicker than the female brain, the adolescent male brain matures less fast than in females making males more likely to take risks. Overall, men are more likely than women to die from suicide, heart disease and from RTAs with excess speed and alcohol contributing to the latter. As adults, money worries, partner problems and uncertainty seem to worry males more than females. Irish men are said to be becoming increasingly vain with 10% admitting that they would consider plastic surgery. Is this a sign of the times or a sign of insecurity?

Women seem to cope better with loss of image, loss of status symbols such as cars or loss of finance whereas these events can turn a man's life upside down. Women are not as dependent on men as they were in their mothers' day and are experiencing more freedom than ever before. Men have not changed in the same way because they have not experienced the same type of change but rather may feel that the traditional male dominance has been undermined. In today's society men may be more vulnerable than in previous times. One third of men surveyed said that they were easily upset by a variety of life events compared to a fifth of women. In a recent series of beer advertisements, men are portrayed as sex-obsessed, incompetent and a joke. Men may now feel that their own status has been reduced to a sexual object to be used and discarded at will. This is worrying and may lead to a serious victimization and undermining of the male status. Better female school and college grades are often highlighted in the media, however men are often skilled at mathematics, science, woodwork, metalwork and environmental studies all of which are extremely important to the economy. While both sexes can be equally good in any subject it is a fact that candidates who are good at either mathematics or science have a wider choice of career opportunity than someone with expertise in the arts.

Autism, Fragile X syndrome, Tourette Syndrome and ADHD occur more commonly in males, possibly because the left side of the brain grows faster than the right side and is more sensitive to increasing testosterone levels, adding to their vulnerability at a young age. Autism is not just one disease but a whole spectrum of conditions often showing withdrawal and a lack of ability to communicate. Autistic individuals may show signs of other problems such as fear or phobias, sleeping and eating disturbances, temper tantrums and aggression. Lack of social interaction persists into adult life. Autism is not confined to childhood. It is found at all IQ levels, those with higher IQ having a better chance of living independent lives. Patients with Asperger Syndrome, a form of autism, are often highly talented and can be quite sociable. Appropriate educational systems can reduce behavioural abnormalities and help coping skills.

Fragile X is the most commonly identified cause of mental handicap. A blood test is diagnostic. It may give rise to a characteristic facial appearance with a long thin face and prominent ears. When one child in the family has Fragile X syndrome there are implications for other family members as this is a genetically inherited condition. Boys who are affected usually have some behavioural and learning difficulties with easy distractability and over-activity. Some subjects may have difficulty relating to other people and special education may be necessary.

Tourette syndrome is a neurological involuntary movement disorder with vocal tics. It begins in childhood or early adolescence and is about 6 times more common in boys than in girls. It has a genetic trigger with different genes associated with different disease manifestations, however there is probably a large environmental component to the disease. Treatment involves behavioural therapy and medication may be useful in some individuals. Tourette syndrome may be associated with obsessive compulsive disorder and ADHD.

Two thirds of subjects with ADHD are boys. ADHD is usually a hereditary condition however alcohol taken in pregnancy may also have a role in its causation. At school, ADHD subjects may find it difficult to concentrate with all the other pupils around, so they become bored. Although ADHD children may still have difficult behaviour and personality as adults they may become high achievers, something to bear in mind when the teacher says that the child is distractible and disruptive. Treatment must put appropriate structures in place to avoid confrontation, to boost self-esteem and to direct the subject into constructive activities. The frustration of dealing with the impulsive behaviour and waiting in hospital for the child to be seen by an expert in the field often with some sense of disappointment at no miracle overnight cure, can lead parents to become abusive. The way to improve a child's behaviour is to ensure that the parents are fair but in control. The internet now offers supervised teaching and correction to disruptive pupils. The appropriate use of stimulant medication is also helpful.

Men are more likely to commit suicide than women. Single men are at greater risk of death. A recent survey indicates that many men in Ireland would like to remain single for as long as possible in order to avoid the expense and time dedication which a family might entail. While this is understandable it is likely that for some men at least, marriage and the family setting offers stability. Social isolation often damages men's health. In the 1960s the annual suicide rate was 64 and suicide in men was rare outside of Dublin. Since 1980 there has been an increase in male suicides from 8 to 18 per 100,000 of the population. Males between the ages of 15 and 24 account for four out of five suicides in Ireland. In 2003 there were 444 suicide deaths registered in Ireland, with the highest suicide rate for five years occurring in men 20-29 years old. In addition, 58 people died from indeterminate causes thought to be suicide-related. More people die in Ireland from suicide than from RTAs. 93% of suicide victims are thought to be suffering from some kind of psychiatric illness. Psychiatric illness seems therefore to have increased substantially since the 1960s. Approximately 18% of men seek psychiatric help prior to a suicide attempt which may involve drowning, poisoning or hanging. Every weekend there are usually at least three deaths from RTAs involving mainly young men, and car crashes are one of the leading causes of deaths in adolescent males who drive with excessive speed on roads not designed for high powered cars. The contribution to RTAs from excess alcohol intake and other drug abuse is substantial. Suicidal ideation in young drivers may well be a further cause. Some GPs are now so distressed over suicide in their practice that they themselves need support. These doctors have indicated that suicide amongst their patients is often impulsive and unpredictable.

Frequently, suicidal subjects suffer from depression but this is often concealed in the male. In order to understand suicide it is necessary to understand depression and how this differs from sadness. Anxiety and despair can be signs of a suicidal tendency. Dedicated time and if necessary antidepressants can give depressed individuals the ability to buy time to address their problems. The Irish in Britain are also more likely to commit suicide than the native population. A coroner in the UK has called the English borough of Camden which has a large Irish community, the suicide capital of England. A lot of these deaths are triggered by alcohol abuse. Low self-esteem is still high amongst Irish people and alcohol is often consumed to cover social and educational inadequacy. Hopelessness and despair have not been adequately addressed despite the increased wealth of Irish society. Suicide prevention programmes enabling earlier detection of vulnerable subjects have begun. Better education and emphasis on reduced alcohol intake must be essential components of such programmes. Young males may be more sensitive than females and may need more interaction from education since they probably find it more difficult to get positive interaction at second-level. A different slant in the Irish school curriculum to address self-esteem problems may be the place to start since high self-esteem would at least make subjects happier and less prone to depression.

The quality of relationships is said to define emotional success in life. Men are often disadvantaged by being seen as the main culprit in marriage breakdown and social or alcohol problems often results in them becoming homeless. The plight of middle-aged separated men often in poor health with very limited resources is a situation that needs remedy by prevention if possible. Recent research in the US indicates that physical abuse of boys by parents at home is common. Alcohol is often the cause of such abuse. Men with a history of physical abuse in the home during their childhood were more likely to be less-well educated than their peers, to be depressed and more likely to get post-traumatic stress. When these boys become men they may repeat the cycle of violence.

More and more Irish people are living in one-parent families. All studies have indicated that dual parenting produces healthier, better educated children so every means possible to avoid social and family disruption must be advocated. Alcohol excess is a frequent cause of family life disruption. Alcohol consumption must be reduced and emphasis on it as part of Irish culture must be removed for good. Excessive time spent at work or in cyberspace can lead to addiction which threatens relationships so it is essential to prevent this addiction before family disruption occurs. Work while at work but make yourself have leisure-time. Get a hobby, talk to your spouse and make time for the children, the cat and or the dog.

The life expectancy of men is less than women however the gap between the two sexes is narrowing. In general men die twice as often as females from heart disease. However all is not doom and gloom because lung cancer is decreasing in males showing that a substantial number of men have given up smoking.

The sexual organs in men are the penis and testes. The testes normally differ slightly in size and shape but if one becomes larger than the other or if a lump develops on the testis, your GP must be consulted to ensure that this is not a cancer. Cancer of the testis though not common has been increasing in incidence in recent years in young men. This has been blamed on environmental oestrogens and other pollutants. The outlook for treatment of this tumour is usually good but it is important to seek advice from the GP as soon as any abnormality is noted. There may soon be a semen screening test for testicular cancer. For everyone's benefit we need to pay attention to the environment and ensure that domestic and industrial waste are disposed off appropriately. Contamination of drinking water can have acute and chronic effects on our health.

Fertility in men may be affected by drinking too much alcohol, by smoking, by eating excessively and by environmental contaminants. In couples with infertility problems, 40% of cases are due to the male partner. Average sperm counts have fallen by more than 50%. This may be due to air pollution or chemicals in the environment. Recent studies have indicated that the quality of men's sperm improved with clean air.

Impotence or inability to get and maintain an erection, can be a problem . This can be a manifestation of general ill health, obesity or diabetes. High blood pressure can be precipitated by eating salty foods and excess alcohol and can contribute to erectile dysfunction. Do not add salt to your food and cut back on alcohol. Intense cycling is great exercise but prolonged periods of cycling on bikes with long narrow saddles can lead to decreased blood flow and numbness in a man's penis. This could lead to impotence. More comfortable saddles should cure this problem. If none of these causes are present and there are no organic reasons for the lack of sexual energy then stress-related reasons may be the cause. For many young men in relationships there is a pressure put upon them by an artificial performance-related culture. Frustration and boredom in relationships can be a problem. An exploration along these lines in a suitable environment may well discover the cause and begin a sexual rejuvenation. For men, dopamine which is a neurotransmitter (transmits signals between brain cells and activates smooth muscle), is said to be the hormone of interest and passion. Dopamine boosters include cottage cheese, low-fat yoghurt, eggs, kidney beans, salmon, cod, ham and liver.

Urinary incontinence is defined as involuntary passage of urine. Male incontinence is unusual before the age of 50 and after the age of 50 it is presumed to be due to prostate problems. In the age group 10-25 years urinary incontinence can be caused by infection, bladder problems or neurological abnormality and needs expert investigation. The prostate gland often enlarges as men get older. This may cause problems passing urine and there is a lot that can be done about this with medication before opting for surgical treatment. Surgical treatment may cause urinary incontinence (lack of bladder control). An implant device may solve or at least improve the incontinence problem.

Approximately one in fourteen men will get prostate cancer and this cancer has been linked to high cholesterol levels. More men die with prostate cancer rather than from it, however vigilance is needed in a patient with a newly diagnosed tumor. A PSA (prostatic-specific antigen level) blood test tends to increase above normal values with prostate cancer. The prostate is examined by a rectal (back passage) examination. Depending on a man's age and on the microscopic appearance on tumor biopsy, it is recommended to have a PSA blood test every 6-12months. If the PSA level is rising, or if the doctor on examination of the prostate gland feels any new areas of growth, then there is reason to suspect that the cancer is advancing and treatment may be indicated. There is now some evidence that the rate of rise of the PSA marker is the important parameter upon which to make a decision for further treatment and more sensitive blood tests are being researched. Radical treatment for prostate cancer can have fairly serious consequences such as urinary incontinence and possible impotence. Androgens are male hormones which tend to stimulate the prostate gland so anti-androgen treatment is useful to inhibit this. The good news is, that in addition to new anti-androgen medical treatment, a new surgical procedure with much less prospect of side effects may soon become available. This combines high frequency ultrasound and laser ablation therapy. Further, while conventional vaccines for children and adults are given to prevent disease rather than treat disease, US researchers have made a vaccine which may help the body to tackle prostate cancer.

Men who lose their hair acutely or gradually are often just as disturbed about this as women. There are quite a few treatments to help males with hair loss so if you are troubled by this you can get help. GPs are often very skilled in this area and will give you whatever advice you need.

Although malignant melanoma is more common in women, men are more likely to die with this because they may neglect to seek help until too late. Men may also be less likely to visit their GPs if these are female. It is important to at least have a GP who you can contact should anything about your health worry you. Educate yourself about the warning signs of health problems. If examination of the genital area causes embarrassment it is always possible to choose a male rather than a female doctor to examine you. Men must become more aware of their own health and seek GP advice if they have health concerns. GPs are able to give very important and sensitive advice on depression, general malaise and cancer affecting the male, particularly on testicular and prostate cancer. If the GP feels that further help for a problem with depression is needed he will be in an excellent position to advise you. For all people, appropriate attention must continue to be made to exercise and acquirement of a hobby, to sensible eating and the avoidance of alcohol excess. The undermining of either sex must not be tolerated in the media, in the home or in society at large.

Key sentences: In a recent series of beer advertisements, men are portrayed as sex-obsessed, incompetent and a joke. This is worrying and may lead to a serious victimization and undermining of the male status. Men must become more aware of their own health and seek GP advice if they have health concerns.

24

Women's Health

Women are not as dependent on men as they were in their mothers' day and are experiencing more sexual freedom than ever before. However, a recent survey has indicated that for Irish women the real pleasure is time spent alone. Pressure at work, in the home and continuous socializing has caused mood swings particularly in the 25-35 year age group. This age group was surprisingly least-focused in the morning. The 55 year and over, age group, was the most content.

Women are more independent than ever, have careers and are able to obtain equal positions in society. The gain in women's independence has however a downside. Women are now beginning to be stressed by work, home and play. While women generally take more care of their health and take note of health warnings, sexual freedom is leading to an increased rate of sexual disease and unfortunately abortions are still occurring. Women's life expectancy used to exceed that for men by 6.5 years however women's life expectancy now exceeds that of a man of similar age by less than five years. This decrease is due to increased binge drinking and smoking in women. Smoking leads to heart disease, lung disease and lung cancer. Heart disease causes many more deaths in women than breast cancer. Cancer of the lung is increasing dramatically in women while the reverse is true for men. There is an increase in liver cirrhosis amongst women with young women regularly binge drinking and putting themselves and a possible future generation of unborn children at severe risk of immediate and long-term health hazards.

ADHD occurrence in children is substantial, possibly due to women drinking alcohol in the early stages of an unsuspected pregnancy. Women because of their smaller size generally become intoxicated quicker and the alcohol tends to be more concentrated than in men. Binge drinking may thus be a factor in the sharp rise of mouth cancer especially in women.

Although America's teenage birth rate is still very high and there is also a high rate of sexually-transmitted disease, teenage girls including African-American girls have now got more assertive and are refusing to have sex. Abortions are down by 40% and abstinence is up. The reverse is true in Europe.

While men are more likely to commit suicide, women are more likely to attempt suicide (parasuicide), mostly with drugs. Fifty percent of female subjects suffer from a psychiatric disorder e.g. depression or alcohol abuse so such subjects should not be left on their own and their medicine chest should be cleared out. The number of women who commit suicide in Ireland has probably increased since 1980 but not to the same extent as men. Irish female suicides in Britain between 1980 and 2000 have also increased. More stable family life and better education, support in the community and from psychiatric services, with reduction of alcohol intake would help to improve this situation.

Whether an overall increased female assertiveness has so undermined the male that the suicide rate in men in Ireland has escalated, is unclear, since female dominance is portrayed both in Ireland and in the UK however the male suicide rate has actually dropped in the UK. It may well be that the change in female status is more dramatic in Ireland since in the seventies and eighties females were a lot more subservient in Ireland compared to the UK. While the status due to women is long overdue it is not appropriate that media advertisements now seem to portray women as the intelligent species while men are often seen as emotional and incapable. Better female school and college grades are often highlighted in the media. While the superiority of these grades must be acknowledged it is also important to stress that many people with good basic education but with very basic grades or none at all have made huge differences to the world. In fact many bosses see a university degree as meaningless and would rather employ someone with good basic education who can read, write, spell correctly and manage money who shows initiative and practical skills. What must be emphasized however is that education of any kind is never wasted, regardless of whether or not a degree or top grade is obtained.

Regardless of how women are portrayed, a lot of Irish women seem to suffer from 'Hurried Woman Syndrome', so priorities need to be established. One cannot be all things to all persons! However much people think that they can 'have it all', they cannot! If you want a career outside of the home adequate provision must be made for appropriate child care. Tasks must be delegated and shared. Family meals must be nutritious whoever cooks them and these should be regular occasions for the family to keep in touch as a unit. Exercise with or without the dog is as important for the female as for the male. This might reduce the need for cosmetic surgery for fat removal in overweight women and would certainly help decrease heart disease which is now a big killer in menopausal women. Smoking must also stop in order to reduce heart disease.

Menstrual period pain is usually self-limiting however it can also be a cause of disability and absence from work. Adequate fluid should be taken in the weeks prior to the event and some non-steroidal anti-pain tablets may also be necessary.

Absence of periods can be psychological, caused by weight loss and strong exercise, chronic illness or by disorders of the ovaries or of the brain. Anti-psychotic drugs may also cause irregularity. It is important to eat sensibly, exercise sensibly and avoid 'pumping iron' to the extreme. Polycystic ovary syndrome (PCOS) is a cause of absence of periods in approximately 7% of pre-menstrual women. Polycystic ovaries are found in families and may be inherited in a dominant fashion. Should periods either not commence or become irregular a visit to the GP will be required.

Failure to ovulate is a cause of infertility. This may be due to PCOS or problems with glands in the head called the pituitary gland or the hypothalamus. Both of these glands regulate hormonal function. PCOS can cause acne, hirsutism and infertility. Hisutism is excessive hair growth on the face and body. Obesity is often present and insulin is secreted in excess. The excess insulin does not cause a low blood sugar because the body is resistant to its effect but it causes male hormones to be secreted in excess from the ovary. Diabetes may also occur. There are quite a few therapies available for PCOS including an anti-diabetic drug which makes the body more sensitive to insulin but does not cause a low blood sugar. This tablet may also help with weight loss. Steroids are used to restore fertility and it is important to remember that pregnancy can occur during treatment.

Our genes and race determine hair growth and in all females, hormonal changes at puberty, during pregnancy and during the menopause can increase hair growth. This usually requires no treatment. Excessive facial or body hair growth can cause physical and psychological problems in women. An abnormal level of hair growth can occur when there is an imbalance of hormones due to problems in the ovaries, the adrenal gland or in the brain. The adrenal gland is in the abdomen and it secretes a variety of hormones. Abnormal hair growth can also occur with certain drugs including the contraceptive pill and steroid medication. Excessive hair growth particularly on the face and chest may be due to disease such as PCOS or other problems in the ovary or adrenal gland. Investigation of excessive facial hair usually involves a series of hormonal tests and may also include imaging of the ovaries or adrenal glands. Depending on the cause of the excessive hair growth, treatment usually involves either electrolysis, tablets containing oestrogen or rarely surgery. PCOS treatment has already been discussed.

In pregnancy some women produce less body hair and may have loss of scalp hair. The hair loss usually recovers after pregnancy.

While in general, men die twice as often as females from heart disease, women of middle age have a greatly increased risk of dying from a heart attack not only because of decreased oestrogen, possible obesity or diabetes but also because of stress. A certain amount of stress before exams or before a public performance may not be a bad thing however excessive and continuous stress is not desirable. Women may be more affected by chronic stress than men and probably form more stress hormones to help cope with the stress. These stress hormones particularly in mid-life may contribute as much to the increase in incidence of heart disease as the decrease in oestrogen.

Obesity is more common amongst women and is an independent risk factor for all causes of mortality. It contributes to a range of poorer health outcomes among women. It is associated with high blood pressure, heart disease, diabetes, menstrual irrregularity, arthritis and gallbladder disease. Being obese also makes you less fertile. The lower the socio-economic status the greater the risk of obesity possibly by the consumption of too much poor-quality food. However it is important not to get over-zealous about weight. Many famous women have aged prematurely and exposed themselves to the risk of osteoporosis and stroke by excessive dieting and over-vigorous workouts. Everyone can look and be healthy by adopting a sensible attitude to food and alcohol with moderate consumption of basic nutritious items, plenty of fruit and vegetables and only occasionally over-indulging in high fat, sugary products. Alcohol consumption should be kept within the limit of 14 units per week. Exercise with sensible eating habits can turn your health around for the better. Smoking is bad for everyone.

Currently, although some areas of the country are carrying out cervical screening programmes there is no national scheme in operation. Bearing in mind that there is a high incidence of sexually transmitted disease and a lower age at commencement of sexual intercourse, both being contributory factors in cervical cancer, nationwide screening should be in place. The traditional screening test is called a Pap test which is done by the GP, in women's clinics and in hospitals. This can successfully detect abnormal cells that lead to cervical cancer. Many women find the procedure uncomfortable and some even avoid the test. Recent research has indicated that women may soon be able to carry out an alternative test at home. This is presently undergoing study trials. It works by microchip technology to measure the electrical resistance in tissues which is altered in the presence of abnormal cervical cells. The microchip is the size of a tampon and can be inserted by the woman herself into the vagina for 10 seconds in order to get a reading. The chip is then sent off for analysis. If trials are successful this test may become available in the next couple of years. A new vaccine against the papilloma virus responsible for cervical cancer is available in the US and this will hopefully have a major impact on the prevalence of cervical cancer.

A recent study has shown that in the A & E department, on average, women were medically assessed thirty minutes after arriving, compared with a twenty minute wait for men. Only 35% of women with heart attacks received thrombolytic (clot-busting) drugs compared to 43% of men. Medical and nursing staff still believe that women have a much lower likelihood of having a heart attack compared to men. The confusion is perhaps understandable by the fact that while men experience typical central chest pain radiating down the arm, women suffering with a heart attack are more likely to experience diffuse pain in the left shoulder with nausea. The message for all medical and nursing staff must be that unfortunately because of obesity and the increase in the number of women smoking, even pre-menopausal women are now almost as likely to have a heart attack as men. Excessive alcohol may also be contributing, by increasing blood pressure. Women and staff must also realize however that there are other reasons for shoulder, chest and arm pain besides heart disease and that with a sensible diet, exercise, avoidance of sexual promiscuity and binge-drinking and by stopping smoking, women can be just as healthy as they want to be!

Key sentences: Women are not as dependent on men as they were in their mothers' day and are experiencing more sexual freedom than ever before. The apparent gain in women's independence has however a downside. Women are now beginning to be stressed by work, home and play.

25

The Older Patient

The older person with vast experience of life can give both children and grandchildren an enormous amount of useful guidance and information. Life expectancy for everyone has increased. Ireland's older citizens now represent the fastest-growing user sector and are becoming more health conscious and more active in their daily lives. While long-stay residential care may be desirable for some older people the vast majority need their own space at home and their independence. 'Telecare' programmes for supporting elderly patients in their own homes will soon be introduced in the UK. Ageing must be a healthy phenomenon. Keeping the mind active by reading, crossword puzzles, chess or card playing is a great way to remain healthy on retirement and is as important as physical exercise. The brain can be improved at any time, regardless of age.

Older women are less likely to receive treatment for cancer than younger women. More comprehensive education for those working with the elderly should change this attitude. The ultimate aim must be to prevent illness. Most people living alone never have any serious problems. Some physical problems such as slow walking speed, osteoarthritis, visual impairment, teeth loss and poorly fitting dentures preventing proper chewing of food, are all more common as people age. Postural problems can also increase with age and sometimes anaesthetic agents used in hospital may cause balance problems to be exacerbated. Falls occur more frequently in the elderly and often lead to fractures (breaks in the bones). Falls may be due to many reasons including:

- poorly fitting shoes,

- bunions and arthritis,

- poor vision,

- dizziness due to heart problems,

- neurological reasons e.g. strokes,

- obesity,

- diabetes,

- poor diet with absence of vitamin D, leading to muscle or bone problems,

- side effects of prescribed or over the counter medication.

45% of all elderly cases that present at A & E are due to falls or blackouts. A confused elderly subject may be misdiagnosed as demented when in fact he has a chronic subdural haematoma which can occur in the elderly after minor head injury. It is essential to try to prevent illness and if possible to avoid falls and fractures which lead to head injury and immobility with all the risks of pneumonia, blood clots and weight gain. Most of the risk factors for falls can be foreseen and should be avoidable by a sensible diet, regular exercise, periodic blood pressure, urine and eye check, and wearing clothes and footwear that are comfortable, warm and easily adjusted. A recent survey has indicated that 40% of X-rays are unnecessary so it is important to avoid inappropriate radiation by keeping healthy and preventing accidents.

Take your time getting out of bed and avoid using cumbersome nightwear. A smoke alarm, good electric wiring and regular servicing of the heating system are essential. Good lighting in the house is extremely important. At Christmas (or any other time) do extinguish any candles or night-lights before bedtime. Always use a proper candle holder and use a heat-proof container for night-lights. Use the handrail every time you use the stairs. Do not carry heavy loads, make several short journeys rather than a marathon! Make sure that no obstacles are obstructing the stairs or passageways. Get any frayed matting or carpet removed.

Good walking shoes must always be worn. A walking stick held in the opposite hand reduces loading on the hip or knee by up to 50%. It is clearly wise to try and prevent falls by the use of hand rails and level floors, by the removal of items that can cause tripping such as trailing wires, loose mats and by good lighting with avoidance of glare and shadow. The routine use of hip protectors cannot be advised as there is no proof that these prevent fractures however they may be considered in some subjects.

Remember that just thirty minutes of exercise per day can reduce the risk of the 'big killers' heart disease, stroke and diabetes. To strengthen bones, weight-bearing exercise is necessary. Walking is an excellent exercise as are bowling, line or ballroom dancing. For those people with mobility problems weight-supported activities such as swimming or cycling are good. Cycling can be a wonderful hobby if you are fit for it and the traffic is not too heavy. Avoid cycling at night or at dusk. It is important to wear a luminous band somewhere on the body if the sky is overcast causing decreased visibility for you and for other traffic. Swimming is a good all-round form of exercise and may also reduce depression, however never go swimming alone . Take extra care if you are taking medication for diabetes or tablets for heart disease or epilepsy. Avoid the risk of getting a stroke by not sprinkling food with salt. There is usually plenty of salt already present in food. Eat at least some fruit and vegetables every day. Avoid vigorous neck movements and have a blood pressure check-up and a blood or urine test for diabetes. A visit to the GP is definitely as important as a visit to the hairdressing salon.

If palpitations occur, get a heart examination with electrocardiogram (ECG). Remember that a heart pacemaker can be acquired, if necessary, at any age. Problems in the thyroid gland which is in the front of the neck, can occur at any age but sometimes are elusive in the older patient. Symptoms can be due to over-activity or under-activity and range from palpitations (rapid heart beat) with weight loss to sluggishness, inability to cope with cold weather and weight gain. A simple blood test can be diagnostic. Do not smoke, particularly if you have asthma or bronchitis. Never smoke in bed!

If you have asthma or bronchitis, always ask your GP for help with the use of an inhaler as he will have several suggestions. All medications being taken should be presented whenever a visit is made to the GP surgery. Always find out why you are taking medications and what each one does to help you. Your GP will be delighted to tell you. If there are severe mobility problems due to arthritis discuss these with your relatives who can help or with your GP who can make arrangements with the district nurse. If your recent eye drops seem to be making your asthma worse this is not your imagination so please discuss with your GP. Medications can have a variety of side effects and can make you forgetful so if you think that you lack your usual intuition since commencing your tablets, talk to your GP about this.

A smoke alarm must be installed on each floor. These are cheap and life-saving. Never forget them!

Make sure that there is a temperature control on the shower. Always check the temperature of the water before showering or bathing. Never use electrical goods in the bathroom. Be familiar with the control knob of the cooker to avoid burns from the hot plates. Turn pot handles inwards but away from the heated cooker plates. Never leave a chip pan, frying pan or grill unattended. A deep fat fryer with thermostat is safer than a chip pan. Do not overuse either! If a fire occurs use a damp cloth or fire blanket to put it out. Make space to rest hot cooking pots to avoid accidental spillage. Get all gas and electrical appliances checked regularly.

Ventilation outlets must never be blocked up. A carbon monoxide detector is an extra precaution. Keep phone numbers of your relatives, friends, GP and local police station near at hand. Keep keys in a safe non-obvious place. Your house or apartment should be made secure with appropriate locks, an alarm and if possible a dog. The dog is the best alarm and he will also ensure that you get daily exercise!

Ask your GP about vaccination against flu and pneumonia and all vaccination necessary if you intend to travel abroad. If you travel to a hot climate watch out for insect bites, too much sun and loosing too much fluid. You may need an insect repellent spray or cream on exposed surfaces, a hat, sunblock and bottled water. If you are travelling to an area where malaria is prevalent you will need to take prophylactic tablets. Two deaths due to malaria, occurred recently in UK travellers who omitted to take these tablets.

It is important to keep informed about the common and some uncommon medical conditions below.

Arthritic pain may be helped by a dietary supplement containing glucosamine sulphate and chondroitin which are the building blocks of cartilage tissue.

Asthma or bronchitis (inflammation of the airways) usually requires an inhaler. The older person may need help to use this. The GP will instruct in its use and often recommends modification of the inhaler with a device called a 'spacer'.

Bone formation and bone maintenance need vitamin D and calcium. Vitamin D is necessary for calcium absorption. Vitamin D can be made in the skin under the influence of sunlight or can be taken in the diet (eggs, cheese, fish). A considerable proportion of vitamin D comes from the effect of sun on the skin which means that in Ireland during the winter months vitamin D stores can be low. Vitamin D deficiency is one of the major causes of bone loss in people who do not go out frequently and eat little vitamin D-containing foods. Vitamins are best taken as part of the diet rather than as supplements however when the diet is deficient or medical conditions exist preventing vitamin absorption, vitamin supplements are necessary. Vitamins should not be over-prescribed since their excess can be harmful and nothing replaces a good healthy diet and exercise.

Hearing tends to wane with age. Many people cannot hear their name being called in the ticket queue or often have to ask friends or relatives to repeat sentences more clearly. There is often an inability to distinguish 's' or 'f'. There may also be ringing in the ear and an intolerance to loud noise. If this is happening to you, see your GP who will examine your ears and your hearing. You may need to have wax removed from the ear. Presbycusis is the deafness that can occur with age. Your GP may need to refer you to a specialist who will prescribe a suitable hearing aid provided there is no reason other than age for the hearing impairment. There are several types of hearing aid depending on where they are worn and the type of technology used. It may take some time to get used to the aid but there will be one that with time will prove of considerable benefit to you. Many people are embarrassed at needing a hearing aid however this is rather foolish as it would be much more embarrassing to miss hearing a speeding car and be knocked down! It is also useful to recall that Ronald Reagan wore a hearing aid and he was known as the 'Great Communicator' so the hearing aid is likely to benefit rather than hinder you.

Incontinence may cause accidental leakage of urine or bowel contents. These conditions can be improved or at least managed in such a way as to avoid embarrassment. Your GP will investigate to find out if there are any serious causes for the incontinence. As a first step make sure that your clothes are comfortable and that going to the toilet does not involve removing several layers of clothes!

There are three main types of urinary *incontinence* called stress, urge and overflow incontinence.

- Stress incontinence means leakage when you cough, sneeze or walk and can be helped by keeping weight down, avoiding smoking and coughing, and practising pelvic floor exercises. The latter can be done in any position and consist of tightening the pelvic floor for as long and as strongly as possible- about 10seconds. Relax in-between and try to do about 10 per day. The same exercise can be done very quickly, holding for just one second and repeated 10 times. Both sets of exercises can be practised about 5 times daily. If you have difficulty with the exercises your GP will help you.

- Urge incontinence causes a sudden need to pass urine. Bladder training helps to control this by gradual lengthening of the time period between visits to the bathroom. If you have difficulty with the bladder retraining, your GP will help you.

- Overflow incontinence means that the bladder does not empty properly and there is constant dribbling. It can be caused by an enlarged prostate, by diabetes affecting the bladder nerves, by Parkinson's disease or even by severe constipation. The underlying condition must be treated. Faecal soiling as well as dribbling is often caused by severe constipation. Make sure that you eat fruit and vegetables to avoid constipation and talk to your GP if the dribbling persists.

Nocturia (Getting up at night to pass urine) decreases quality of life. Prostate problems in men and loss of urinary control in women can become troublesome as we age however both can be helped by talking to your GP regarding medication for men and pelvic exercises for women.

Shingles is a painful rash usually on one side of the face or body, caused by the chickenpox virus which after many years may become reactivated. It occurs most frequently in the elderly and is called herpes zoster. One cannot get shingles from someone with chickenpox but one can get chickenpox from someone with shingles. People with shingles should therefore avoid pregnant women or young children who have not had chickenpox or people with susceptibility to infection because of other illnesses or immune deficiency. Early signs of shingles before the rash appears include, pain, tingling, aching or numbness, on one side of the body. It is important to see your GP as soon as possible because the drug that he will prescribe for you is a substance called aciclovir, which will only work if it is started within 2-3 days of the rash appearing. This drug is useful for preventing permanent scars from the rash and will relieve the pain. Sometimes shingles causes the pain to return about three months after the rash and this can happen even if the aciclovir was given in time. Your GP will be able to prescribe some other tablets to relieve the pain. He will advise you regarding the best clothes to wear to stop the pain irritating the skin – usually loose cotton underwear and loose outside clothes. If the pain continues, your GP may refer you for transcutaneous electrical nerve stimulation (TENS). A vaccine against shingles has become available in the US and this has been shown to reduce the burden of illness caused by herpes zoster .

Everyone needs new scenery from time to time and *travel* for the older person should hold no barriers. It is important however to be aware of the dangers of extreme environmental conditions such as hot climate and high altitude. If you have a heart or lung problem consult your GP before flying as a recent study indicates that oxygen levels during flights can drop to lower values compared with ground levels. In some cases this change might precipitate angina although it should pose few problems unless serious heart or lung problems are present. While the older person is unlikely to take up mountain climbing in later life, it is important to be aware that flying straight without a stop-over to destinations over 3000 metre height above sea level (places in South America), may not be wise. Symptoms of high altitude sickness can begin at 2000 metre so a slow gradual rate of ascent is desirable. Symptoms of acute mountain sickness vary from headache, nausea, dizziness, chest tightness or breathlessness to loss of balance, drowsiness and disorientation.

Travel by boat although slower than a plane journey can be very calming and enjoyable however motion sickness can be very sickening and a problem at any age until one gets regular exposure to ferry travel. Travel by hovercraft is not ideal if the seas are choppy. It is essential to eat very little before travelling. Sit up on deck if possible. Close the eyes to avoid looking at moving objects. Avoid reading and try and limit head movement. Medication may be necessary. Motion sickness is not common on trains.

Blood clots in the legs can occur with prolonged immobility so while travelling on the boat, train or plane get up occasionally and if possible walk around, drink some water and avoid alcohol. Talk to your doctor regarding the use of aspirin pre-travel. Do not sit for prolonged periods in the car. Stop and walk around in a suitably safe place.

Research in Ireland has indicated that older bus passengers suffer most in non-collision accidents occurring while boarding and alighting from the bus. It is always wise to take preventive measures and if possible avoid peak traffic travelling when time pressure may cause the driver to take off and stop at top speed. It is also wise for those who have any mobility problems to avoid climbing stairs in buses.

The use of public transport is recommended for all, including the older person. However the ability to drive is often important for the social functioning of the older patient. It is essential that all drivers are medically fit to drive for their own protection and for that of the public. At any age, problems with dizzy sensations or loss of balance such as vertigo should be sorted out before driving.

Vision needs regular assessment. As one ages, glasses for reading are usually required. An eye test every two years is wise after age 65 years. Tell-tale eye signs may predict a stroke and therefore eye examination may help to prevent the stroke occurring. Examination of the eye may reveal not just an eye problem but a general medical problem such as diabetes which unfortunately is common and needs diagnosis and treatment as soon as possible. In the older age groups particularly, vision may deteriorate due to cataract, macular degeneration or glaucoma. Cataract causes the lens to cloud over. Cataract is easily managed. The eye specialist will advise regarding surgery to the eye, and subsequent use of glasses or a contact lens. There are several types of contact lens and the optometrist will advise regarding their suitability for each individual.

Macular degeneration is a retinal condition where cells at the centre of the retina degenerate causing a big deterioration in vision. Some forms of *macular degeneration* may be treatable if detected early and recent research suggests that a good diet with adequate fresh fruit and green vegetable intake can help prevent some forms of macular degeneration. Foods that may help the eye include spinach, broccoli, corn, kale and tomatoes or tomato sauce. Recent research suggests that new technology may allow a tiny telescope to be implanted in the eye in order to enlarge images and reduce the blind spot in macular degeneration.

Chronic glaucoma is a condition occurring in the eyes which gradually leads to a loss of vision by increased eye pressure. It tends to run in families and can occur particularly in people who are short-sighted, in diabetic patients, in patients with circulatory disorders and with increasing age. If there is a family history of glaucoma, family members should have an eye check-up. Acute glaucoma is even more damaging to the eye than chronic glaucoma and occurs most frequently in the elderly. It is characterized by sudden onset of pain around the eyes or an ache around the brow, with blurring of vision. Vomiting may occur. Prompt treatment is necessary to save the sight in the eye. It is important to be aware that glaucoma may occur for no apparent reason or may be secondary to other causes such as injury, blood clot or haemorrhage in the eye. Acute glaucoma can also follow the use of eye drops which have been put in the eye in order to dilate the pupil for eye examination. Glaucoma is treated with special eye drops but occasionally surgery may be needed to reduce the pressure in the eye.

Since treatment for cataracts and glaucoma is usually very effective it is mandatory that the senior members of the household do not deteriorate in an unnecessary twilight zone.

Key sentence: Ageing must be a healthy phenomenon.

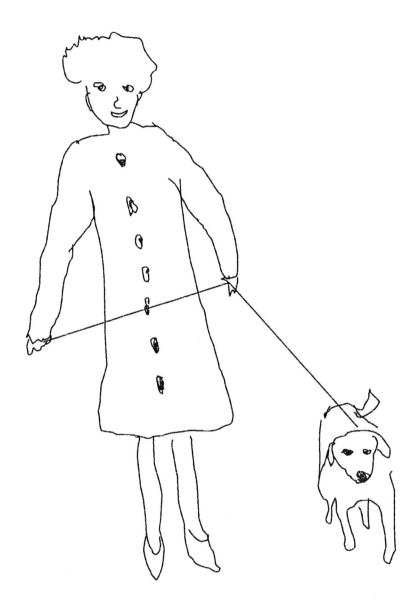

I AM A HAPPY, ACTIVE AND HEALTHY OCTOGENARIAN

Table 1

Acceptable ranges of weight at various heights. The higher end of range being more likely in males.

Height /metre*	feet	inches	Weight (kg)	(stone)	BMI
1.48	4	11	42-54	6.6-8.5	19-25
1.50	5	0	45-58	7.1-9.1	20-26
1.53	5	1	46-59	7.3-9.3	20-25
1.55	5	2	47-61	7.4-9.6	20-25
1.58	5	3	51-64	8.0-10.0	21-26
1.60	5	4	52-66	8.2-10.4	20-26
1.63	5	5	54-68	8.5-10.7	20-26
1.65	5	6	57-71	9.0-11.2	21-26
1.68	5	7	58-72	9.1-11.3	21-26
1.70	5	8	59-74	9.3-11.6	20-26
1.73	5	9	60-76	9.4-11.9	20-25
1.75	5	10	62-79	9.7-12.4	20-26
1.78	5	11	64-82	10.1-12.9	20-26
1.80	6	0	66-84	10.4 -13.2	20-26
1.83	6	1	68-86	10.7-13.5	20-26

*Height without shoes
1 kg = 2.2 pounds
14 pounds = 1 stone
1 foot = 0.3 metre

References:
- Textbooks of Medicine
- Media

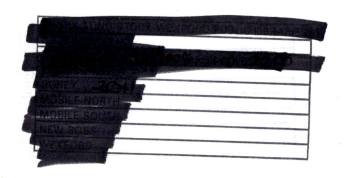

Printed in the United Kingdom
by Lightning Source UK Ltd.
127701UK00001B/31-33/A